After Fortune Green

AFTER FORTUNE GREEN

Fred Nailer

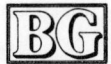

The Book Guild Ltd
Sussex, England

The Book Guild Ltd.
25 High Street,
Lewes, Sussex.

First published 1991
© Fred Nailer 1991
Set in Baskerville

Typesetting by Kudos Graphics
Slinfold, Horsham, West Sussex
Printed in Great Britain by
Antony Rowe Ltd.,
Chippenham, Wiltshire.

British Library Cataloguing in Publication Data
Nailer, Fred
    After fortune green.
    1. Polyomyelitis victims – Biographies
    I. Title
    362.1968350092

ISBN 0 86332 540 8

CONTENTS

DEDICATION

To my wife, Enid Mary, who has made life not only possible but also a great joy for me on the scale detailed in the following chapters.

1

Fortune Green

My father was born in a house in Cholmeley Road, Reading, by the cemetery, in 1893, and my grandparents moved to London around the turn of the century, where their new home was at West Hampstead on the ground floor of a three storey terrace house near Fortune Green. My grandfather, Fred I, collapsed and died on the site of St. John's Wood Power Station in 1907 and as the years rolled by, my father went to France and returned to join the GPO as a postman wearing one of those little flat topped hats like a truncated policeman's helmet.

Achilles Road was on the poor side of West End Lane and across the lane rose those gentle slopes towards Hampstead Heath and the larger homes where domestic help was employed. The postman's walk took my father around these streets of Frognal and there he met a domestic helper whom he married in Fulham in 1924.

Not by choice did I arrive just after the General Strike – there being no possible connection – in that terraced house of a Victorian street off Fortune Green, West Hampstead.

In my young life the Sunday morning constitutional was to be pushed by my father in that very deep perambulator with smallish wheels, from Achilles Road to Hampstead Heath, but photographic evidence is the only memory of the many perambulations along Spaniards Road and across the Heath and the few live memories of that time include the neighbour calling to enlist the services of my grandmother by saying,

'It's Mr. Fensome, will you come and have a look at him. We think he has died!'

What purpose this inspection served always mystified me!

7

At the bottom of the small garden, a ladder or frame was built for me to climb up to see over the fence to the 'boys' home' in the next street. Some sort of institution for naughty boys that always had me slightly worried by its grim appearance.

In the summer of 1930 we moved to Metroland, to a new house on the original development of the Chalkhill Estate at Wembley Park. A house all to yourself, a third acre plot with a hundred yards of back garden that seemed so enormous to a four year old, but it stretched down to the railway that was to prove such a source of interest in later life.

At the bottom of the garden the Metroland railings were at the foot of a grassy bank with ornamental trees to shield the residents from the horrors of the railway. So you retreated up the garden and eventually up the stairs to the back bedroom windows where you could survey a vast, and very interesting panorama of activities. Hard by on the left was Neasden Power Station and all the women muttered mightily about the smuts descending from these tall chimneys on to their washing, but the great timber cooling towers and all that steam were very impressive to a small boy – I could not think why they worried about their stupid washing. The defunct Wembley Exhibition occupied most of the due south aspect with the mighty British Government Pavilion on the skyline gazing westwards towards the Stadium – the largest structure for miles around.

Many other exhibition buildings were visible, either derelict or in their new uses such as the 'Magicoal Fires' building or the more mysterious 'UKANSEE' where it was fondly believed they made cellophane paper. In the foreground was a shedlike building that really went unnoticed until the night in 1931 when it caught fire and the flames lit the night sky, bringing the Wembley Urban District Council Fire Brigade out in force to end the life of a wireless factory.

Right across the foreground was visible a good half mile stretch of Metropolitan Railway tracks offering lots of interesting happenings and beside them the Great Central trains appeared at infrequent intervals; further away the High Wycombe line trains climbed towards Wembley Hill and disappeared behind the British Government Pavilion and sweeping round to the foreground was the Stadium loop where a motley selection of trains served Stadium Station on Cup Final days. It was on Cup Final day in 1931 that my interest in the Stadium loop was diverted to a far greater attraction by the chugging along right overhead of the Graf Zeppelin, the biggest and slowest thing I had ever seen. It trundled along with the gondolas clearly visible and passed so low over the stadium that I feared for the flags flying from stubby poles around the top of the walls.

The weekly 'must' came on Sunday mornings when the locomotive shed and the little coaling stage of the Metropolitan all came to life and there was a great shunting in and out of all the weird collection of motive power on the shed. There were more than thirty locomotives on the shed in those days from the two little Peckett saddle tanks that seldom seemed to appear, to the E and F classes, and one or two of the original Class As. All these were mixed in long lines with the big tank engines with the deep steam hooters that plyed passenger and goods trains down the line as they were each in turn cleaned, coaled and watered for work on Monday morning.

The tarmac surface of Barnhill Road itself ceased two doors away and the rest was an unmade road that still tempted a lot of drivers to try this short cut avoiding the climb over Blackbird Hill. A few yards from the end of the tarmac surface there was a constant puddle that absorbed many a rear wheel that had to be towed out again. The most spectacular effort was a big three axle Sentinel Steam Wagon whose nearside rears sank deep into the puddle and remained there for a couple of days until another mighty huffing monster of its kind arrived to provide the weight and the power to move the stricken steamer from the mire.

Wembley Park Station was the focal point of transport and many journeys were made in the Ashbury Stock and the clerestory roofed saloons, usually to Baker Street, to climb the stairs and descend to the westbound Inner Circle for journeying on to Kensington High Street Station in Ponting's arcade. Out into the High Street to the bus stop to wait for a No. 28, and when it came along, the driver might just lean out from what there was of a cab on a NS bus and say, 'Hello, son'. It would be my grandfather, David Harper, a driver with the General since horse bus days.

Visiting his home in Fulham, I remember being taken on a

bus ride. Climbing to the open top deck, sitting on the wooden seats and when the conductor came round, my grandpa would produce this photograph of himself in uniform and all question of fare payment for him or myself seemed to be overlooked and we were immediately great mates with the conductor. It was on one of these trips that I was marched out from home dressed in a black velvet suit as part of the ceremonial of my Aunt Winifred's wedding, a suit that I managed to evade ever wearing again and that I wore only very reluctantly on that occasion.

Walking up that little road in Fulham, with its terrace houses, each with a little bay window, three feet back from the coping stones on the low wall that was surmounted with ornamental railings, a wooden wheelchair stood in that space at a house across the road. There was always a man sitting in that chair in front of that little house, but at that age I had difficulty in working out what it was all about, but of course, you learn!

About this time I was introduced to the motor car when my father gave up as an insurance agent and took to fishmonger- ing. We acquired a 7 hp 1927 Jowett tourer and collected a consignment of boxes of wet fish at Wembley Park Station every morning. The fish came by train overnight from Grimsby and out on the Metropolitan to our home station. My father was not a particularly accomplished driver having had lessons from my grandfather, who only knew how to drive a bus. There being no driving examination in those days, all seemed to be well if you could steer clear of impact, which mostly we did.

Early days at school led on to the summer holidays in 1933 and my first visit to Broad Oak, a large modern house built by one Ernest Evans, on a ten acre woodland site in Hatch Lane, Bucklebury. A full plumbing service was fitted up with bath, basins, sink and flush toilets, all served from a header tank filled from a well by hand pump, there being no electricity in the neighbourhood to provide power or lighting, for which oil lamps were provided. Ernie Evans was a cousin, by marriage, of my father and Bucklebury village school had tutored a considerable number of Nailers long before John Nailer married Mary Anne Wigmore and produced a large family there in the 1800s.

Broad Oak was built in 1930, a big double fronted house in clean pink brickwork, with an arched porch to the front door, that led to a wide hallway extending through the house to the back door. On the lefthand wall of the hallway, a straight staircase led to a balcony around three sides of the lofty hall, from which all four bedrooms were accessible.

At the head of the stairway on the left was the bathroom with all mod cons of the age and water supplied by the hand pump in the kitchen to the roof storage tank on which string was attached to a float arm that led down through the floors to the kitchen, whence a plumb bob on the end of the string gauged the water level in the tank against markings on the wall. I always felt that the size of the tank must be considerable, as my efforts on the pump handle could only ever move that plumb bob an imperceptible degree.

On the ground floor with the hall and the kitchen were only three other rooms, the left hand front being the largest with a French window in the side wall leading to the garden. Sash windows with large panes were all round the house including the two front bays and in the gable ends, the roof had opening porthole windows.

In the corner of the hall by the front door stood a grandfather clock on which rested a blue spiked helmet retrieved from some unfortunate German soldier during Ernie's service in France! A range of paraffin lamps stood around the house although I do not remember the cooking arrangements as I was more interested in the eating procedures.

Later development saw another doorway built at the back of the upstairs balcony and a narrow stairway leading forwards up into the attic and encroaching on the ample back bedroom space. The attic space was partitioned off to make two colossal rooms which remained essentially attic space, although the portholes gave way to larger sash windows at that time. To sleep up here was of course, a boy's delight, although when the house was full, as it often was, I can't ever remember queueing for the bathroom, so perhaps my washing was frugal and anyway, there was another loo under the verandah outside the back door.

The general air of Broad Oak was space in those sunny summer days in the Thirties but in the long dark days of winter, out of sight of the lane which was about 100 yards away, it could well have been less inviting.

A rough timber garage stood in a layby along the driveway and another later development was a substantial brick built garage attached to the right hand wall of the house. This garage had a 'round the corner' sliding door that was an intriguing arrangement to me and behind the garage, a tank or reservoir collected all the rainwater from the roof of the whole house and the garage. These were the needs of the age!

The most interesting place to me was the workshop – an old army hut in sections placed end to end and to walk through there was to imagine a clerestory roof and all the seats of saloon stock on the Metropolitan. In reality there were benches, racks, tools, jigs and building material that were the stock in trade of the owner and to wander through section after section was always to see something new in preparation such as the pair of heavy timber gates that always stood open at the end of the drive, shining white, as an example of the work of Ernie Evans. Those gates still stand nearly 60 years after, but in a sadly neglected state.

John Nailer was one of six children of William Nailer who farmed in Bucklebury in the early nineteenth century. John became the father of thirteen children, all born in Bucklebury and this included more than one set of twins. My grandfather Frederick was one of the children, born in 1862, but the only members of that generation that I knew were at the younger end of the line. Alfred lived in the thatched cottage on the Common – the Avenue – and collapsed and died outside the front gate in 1940. Aunt Tilly was the youngest and a twin, and she lived in Beenham, while Aunt Liz lived with Ernie and Lilly Evans, being Aunt Lil's mother. I was once taken to see Aunt Betsy in an upstairs room of a tiny thatched cottage between Chapel Row and the village of Bucklebury. She lay abed and was considerably bloated and hushed whispers were to be heard of 'dropsy'!

The stay at Broad Oak was the highlight of my year; free to tear around those acres of woodland and swing high into the branches of a big oak tree not far from the house. A self–employed builder and decorator, Ernie was a motorist before the 1914 war and on my first visit to Broad Oak, he drove us away from Reading Station in a large lumbering Singer

Tourer, with all over hood and flapping celluloid side screens. You climbed on to the running board and then up into the car to sit beside the driver, where all the action was. Out on the long sweeping bends of the Bath Road beyond Theale in the Singer was an exhilarating experience, before you turned off up Cod's Hill and past Douai Abbey towards Hatch Lane.

It was here in Bucklebury that I had my one and only ride in a pony and trap with Great-Uncle Alf and so the holiday passed by and Broad Oak was but a memory until the following summer when drought struck hard in these rural parts served only by well water. In August 1934 I had four weeks at Broad Oak amid the water shortage and at one stage a horse-drawn water cart arrived and the contents were discharged into the well to be hand pumped – sparingly – up into the roof tanks.

In Jubilee Year there were trips to London to see the new fangled flood lighting of County Hall, Shell Mex House and other stately buildings; rides on the trams through the tram subway from Victoria Embankment and a visit to Baker Street to see King George and Queen Mary ride by in an open landau on one of their ceremonial drives round London. Not that royalty were anything new to me, as my grandmother always marched me out on Cup Final days to be in the front row of the crowd that gathered to see the Royal Patronage drive by on the approach to Wembley Stadium, for the formal presentation of the cup.

I celebrated the Jubilee itself in bed with scarlet fever, but as an only child I was permitted to stay at home surrounded by a new disinfectant on the market as recommended by the doctor – Dettol!

Six weeks away from school was wonderful but bed was a little boring at 8½ years old and it was not helped on St. George's Day when my mother arrived with glad tidings.

'What do you think your Auntie Winnie has got?' she said.

My mind turned to the little wire haired terrier that she kept. 'Another dog?' I said.

'No' was the emphatic reply.

I pressed on with canaries, tortoises, budgerigars, cats, monkeys and parrots, but the denials were becoming increasingly less patient.

Then my mother said triumphantly 'She's got a little boy!'

I failed to respond with any kind of enthusiasm which proved a great disappointment to my mother and she brushed aside the Dettol sprinkled curtain that hung over the doorway and departed downstairs.

No other children were ever born into the near family in that generation so perhaps I should have been more chivalrous, but babies did not impress at the age of 8½.

It was about this time that I began to realise the great information value of the common cigarette card, for they told you about the things you were really interested in – so unlike the much vaunted encyclopedias. Motorcars, aeroplanes, warships, the faces of the voices that were heard on the radio and the imagined faces of the Kings and Queens of England from the year dot. All these cards carried a wealth of detail on the subject depicted, although I never really could arouse much interest in film stars, wild flowers or fish. This magical source of knowledge was put to good use one afternoon on the school playing field when a small circle of us stood and gazed up at a dark painted twin engined aeroplane climbing away from Hendon Aerodrome, at a speed scarcely greater than the Zeppelin. We stood in awed silence and a voice in the circle said 'It's a night bomber'. It was a Fairy 'Hendon', the latest thing of the day.

On another occasion we were standing at the school gate surveying a rather tatty 10 hp Austin Saloon with two men inside and my companion murmured confidentially

'It's a "Q" car and they are policemen, and under the bonnet is a Bentley engine!"

My own fond visions of a Bentley engine told me there was hardly the space aboard and anyway, the weight would crush those rusty wire wheels.

There was an unexpected summons to the school assembly hall one afternoon and when all were foregathered, the headmaster addressed us in very sombre tones which evolved as a lecture on the evils of dishonesty. Adopting the 'this will hurt me more than it will hurt you' approach, he went on to lay bare the detected crimes of three school pupils. They had stolen a pump and a cycle lamp from a bicycle and each received six hefty whacks across the buttocks before the entire school. We were all very impressed, particularly the three culprits.

The headmaster was a kindly man with some futuristic ideas and this led to the formation of a gardening class. A chunk of the playing field was dug up, horticultural specimens were planted, crazy paving paths laid out and we made a concrete birdbath to instructions, but the most interesting job was the lawn-mower and this duty fell to myself and a friend on numerous occasions. We would extract the mower from the store room, lay the cast iron wheels on the concrete floor of the corridor and push. The ensuing noise brought doors open on all sides and angry heads popped out to protest, so we picked up the mower and fled to the garden.

When Grandpa came to retire from the buses at this time, another valuable source of information dried up; the regular supply of TOT ('Trains, Omnibuses and Trams') which became Pennyfare, the staff magazine of London Transport. From these pages I made a scrapbook of vintage pictures and the stories of new works programmes, the new rolling stock for the railways, the building of the world's largest trolley bus fleet and the planned demise of the tramcar in London.

On my ninth birthday, we had a trip to Southend on an Eagle Steamer from Tower pier. The 'Crested Eagle' was a paddle steamer and you could walk round below deck and see all the highly polished machinery that turned the paddle wheels as it worked. The 'Crested Eagle' survived for another five years before being sunk at Dunkirk. Coronation year was another great celebration and in Wembley all the school children were taken to the new Empire Pool to a special performance of a circus and in the Stadium, serried ranks of girls in black drawers and white blouses did 'knees bends' and the rest, under the waving arms of Prunella Stack. The Women's League of Health and Beauty was with us and as a rather more exciting attraction, the Chrysler Hell Drivers did all the things that Hell Drivers usually do in the Stadium arena.

In 1938 I ploughed through my eleven plus examination and gained a place at a secondary school and there was a letter from Broad Oak to say that Ernie was selling up and would we like to go for a last holiday there? Would we just!

We were met at Reading Station by Ernie now driving a 1930 Austin 12/4 with chromium radiator surmounted by a

circular thermometer but still with the all over hood and
celluloid side screens. On Saturday afternoon we drove the
twelve miles back into Reading to meet my father arriving on
an afternoon train and on the way we were almost involved
in a whimsical accident, when one of the Corporation open-
topped four-wheeled tramcars stopped at traffic lights causing
the following Royal Mail van to brake quite suddenly. Alas
for the brand new Austin Ruby 7, which struck the back of
the mail van quite forcibly to leave its headlamp glasses in the
road, but our elderly tourer just managed to pull up short of a
further collision. The tram moved off, the mail van passed the
cross roads and pulled in, the Ruby pulled in before the cross
roads and Ernie Evans, a very restrained and sober man,
pressed the tourer away up the road at speed round the
outside of the tram, which drew the postman's attention so
that he climbed back into his van and gave chase. As we
nipped round a series of left and right hand turns, my mother
and my aunt in the back seats were peering out of the
celluloid peephole and yelling,

'He's coming round the corner, Ernie'. We drove into the
triangular car park at the end of Thorn Street and as we all
got out of the car, the postman marched menacingly into the
car park and accused Ernie of ramming his mail van. A
debate ensued and the postman examined the dumb irons
and the wing tips of the Austin for damage, but not a mark
was to be found. He took our names and addresses and then
turned to me. 'Sonny Evans?' he queried. 'No', I said
indignantly, 'Sonny Nailer'. He walked away, a very saddened man as he realised he had been taken for a ride.

This was one last wonderful carefree holiday at Broad Oak
and a visit to the old thatched cottage on the Avenue of
Bucklebury Common where we were photographed with
pitchforks for imaginary haymaking. Just how significant that
photograph would be was not realised at the time or when we
first reached home.

The days of Fortune Green had almost run out.

2

The Birthday Present

All summer in 1938, the newspapers had given names and ages of folk who had died in the polio wave and this left the impression in my mind that no one ever survived with polio. Nothing was further from my mind on one of my last days at Junior School when I followed a friend of mine home via a mucky alley along the back of the churchyard, where a dirty wet ditch wound its way down to the River Brent.

Home from my holiday and measured for a new school uniform for my first term at Preston Manor School, I began to feel unwell and was put to bed. Eventually the doctor was called and nothing was said, but he called again the next day, by which time I had been out of bed and stood up, but one foot remained under the bedclothes as I could not bring it to the floor below me. My father drew it out and placed it where it should be, but I had other troubles too; I was quite unable to pass water.

'Rheumatism,' they told me. 'You will have to go into hospital for a few days.'

I was a little puzzled by this but I felt distinctly unwell and my over-riding desire was to relieve the pressure on my bladder, which increased with the passage of time. On Friday, the dark blue fever ambulance arrived from Acton and I was loaded aboard with my mother and father. The driver set off for the RNO Hospital at Stanmore but obviously had little idea of where to go, so we drove around seemingly endlessly while my bladder pressure increased along with my father's anxiety about the driver ever finding Stanmore, let alone the hospital, but eventually we did arrive and I was put to bed in an isolation room on Surgical Ward, so named because it was adjacent to the operating theatre. The bed had a water-filled mattress on a fracture board and every slight movement I was able to make was accompanied by a surging and glug-glugging of the water contained in a mattress shaped red rubber cover rather like a great big inner tube of a pneumatic tyre.

I was interviewed at length by the houseman who wrote down my life history long–hand, that remains on the file to this day. Somewhere along the line I was given some strange concoction to drink from a very chipped enamel feeding cup and almost immediately I enjoyed great and voluminous relief of the bladder.

Unknown to me I was really very seriously ill and I remember only one thing for the next week and that is waking at night in this long, narrow and very dark room to find I was completely alone and I gave vent to my disturbed state by exercising my lungs, long and loud, before eventually a ginger–haired nurse appeared who told me to be quiet and go back to sleep. This I eventually did, still alone in the pitch dark of this very strange room. The effects of this incident were soon to show on my health. They told me that visitors came on Sunday, but all this remains a blank in my memory as do all the developments during Sunday night which were afterwards related to me by Mr John Cholmeley, a resident orthopaedic surgeon and a Fellow of the Royal College.

Perhaps I am fortunate that someone noticed signs of respiratory failure that night, which prompted a lot of telephone activity to locate an available mechanical respirator which was eventually found at the Hospital for Sick Children in Great Ormond Street, WC2.

'You will need a furniture van and six men to move it', said Great Ormond Street.

'Don't bother', was the reply, 'We'll come to you, stand by!'

The details of this story were related to me by John Cholmeley FRCS on an occasion many years later as I was being 'plastered' by this surgeon for a replacement leather moulded corset as part of the structural steelwork that held body and soul together. The technique here was to encase the body in a thick layer of plaster bandages with a two inch strip of lead beneath the plaster from the Adam's apple to the penis and with the plaster well moulded to the body and setting, a large pointed knife is applied to the plaster at chest level and drawn vigorously downward to cut through the plaster on to the lead strip. Thoughts of any consequences of that sharp knife point running off the lead strip or failing to stop before grounding on the bench beneath the buttocks, is cause for grave concern and apprehension by the male patient.

The plaster cast is then parted at the front, removed from the body and brought together again for binding with more plaster bandage to form in itself a mould for the manufacture of a solid plaster 'body' around which the boot leather corset can be moulded. But to return to the night of Sunday 14 August 1938. . .

Thus it was that Mr Rice, the hospital maintenance engineer, was dragged from his bed to drive the hospital ambulance, a large modern and very stately Austin vehicle finished in a hideous shade of yellow with the orthopaedic symbol emblazoned on the sides and all mounted on fat low pressure tyres of the age. With the patient loaded in the ambulance, the driver at the helm and Mr Cholmeley and Mr Seddon – to become Professor and later Sir Herbert Seddon – effecting artificial respiration on the patient, we set off from Stanmore for Great Ormond Street.

This part of the venture was successfully accomplished although I was taking little interest at the time or when I was loaded into the Drinker, so called after the American designer, Philip Drinker, but dubbed by the popular press as an 'Iron Lung'. This large coffin-shaped box on legs had a full length tray in the bottom and a plate forming the head end of the box was attached to this tray, so that the tray could be slid out of the box, the patient placed on the tray as a bed and his head would be forced through a large sorbo rubber ring in the head plate. Then the tray or bed would be closed into the box, the head plate clamped air tight to the box, leaving only the patient's head in view. A cumbersome electric pump did all the huffing and puffing of artificial respiration in the air tight box, in the sides of which were port holes with some kind of built-in seal through which the nursing staff could operate should the need arise.

The whole contraption was painted dark green and there

was a nurse in constant attendance. By day there was Nurse Bispham and by night, it was Dilys Jones, who watched over me, but still I took little interest in them or the rest of the world, although some of the rest of the world was beginning to take an interest in me, as was evidenced by the arrival, a day or two afterwards, of a photographer from the *Daily Express*. I was then becoming slightly aware of the goings on around me and there were a few short trial openings of the Drinker which I somehow survived. On the fourth day, Thursday 18 August, there was another trial opening of the machine and I was lifted out on to a bed alongside. This was my twelfth birthday and I seemed to be the object of a great deal of attention from a number of apparently important people whom I had never seen before.

Among the procession there came a stately lady whom I later discovered to be the Matron and her words to me that day were prophetic.

'This is the best birthday present you will ever have, my boy', she said and my mind immediately went to the selection of purchaseable items that I had hoped to receive on my birthday. It was a long time before the significance of that lady's words really registered with me, but I know now that I have had cause to remember them thankfully over the years.

On the site where my father was employed, the foreman made up the wage packets each week and this particular week there was an extra shilling piece wrapped in a small piece of paper on which it said 'For the boy'. One of many kind thoughts at that time.

Nurses J Bispham and Dilys Jones continued their day and night surveillance over me and who should roll up again but the man from the *Daily Express*. He arrived on a Sunday afternoon at visiting time, which displeased me and the following day there I was on the back page of the *Daily Express* amid a full page of world news pictures. There were two photographs of myself, one showing the Drinker with my head sticking out and reflected in the driving mirror above – this gave the patient a slightly more extended view of the room and the nurses – and the second picture, taken on that Sunday afternoon showed me with my arms above my head 'waking up in the morning'.

Newspapermen always love the dramatic approach, true or otherwise, and perhaps this is why they had always been so keen to spread the despondency of the mortality rate among those who contracted polio without mention of those who recovered, albeit disabled. That despondency which had troubled me earlier that summer had at last been put in true perspective in a national daily.

The appearance of these pictures with my name and the hospital address brought a selection of correspondence mostly telling me that I was a 'poor, brave boy', which is nonsense. Bravery comes when you have the choice of pressing on or running away and although I was quite enjoying my new found importance, not feeling too bad and being exceedingly well cared for, by choice I would still have run away home from the whole business. Disability is one of the things that comes your way in life and you have to get on with it as best you can with whatever help you are fortunate enough to have around you.

Not all the letters however, were like this. One that came from Bishopsthorpe near York was from a schoolboy asking if he could write to me while I was in hospital. Over the years, Francis Stirk fell foul of rheumatic fever eventually becoming a resident in the Cheshire Home at Alne Hall in Yorkshire and we corresponded for many a long year on each Friday the 13th. It was about this time also, an uncle of mine, Cyril Porter, with fellow feeling for disability, began writing me the occasional letter to brighten my hospital stay. His fellow feeling came from a cycling accident that led to the development of spondylitis, an arthritic condition of the spine that caused spine and hips to solidify making walking and sitting down extremely difficult. This letter led to an ultimate regular correspondence which was spurred on by his first letter suggesting that when I last visited their home in Wimbledon, I had tied a knot in the cat's tail and the cat was not very pleased about it. I bit very hard on this one and made frantic denials that it was me. How that cat must have suffered!

By this time the Munich crisis was with us and there were great changes in the medical arrangements at the hospital due to some senior American staff leaving for home on the Queen Mary but we were getting down to the extent of my paralysis which was total from the waist down without the flicker of a toe, the water works still did not and punitive measures were being taken to alleviate the strain on the bladder. On the credit side, the respiratory problems seemed to be solved and there was full use in my arms, shoulders and hands; we are just getting clear of the infection period and my one desire is to see that I am home in time to visit Gamages before Christmas.

The care of a patient at Great Ormond Street was superb; pressure points rubbed with meths and powder every four hours, day and night, modest physiotherapy that prevented dropped feet, kept all the joints free of stiffening up and saw to it that I remained the correct general shape, which is one of the major problems with polio in children.

There were balconies all round the building and in the autumn sunshine, you could be wheeled out in your bed to have a better view of the roof tops of London, which included a distant sight of a church dome which I thought was St Paul's and it may well have been, but I could not work out how I could possibly see St Paul's from Stanmore, as I was still not fully aware of how I had been moved to the HSC. Another balcony view was the winch lorry in a nearby square that launched and winched in a barrage balloon, one of a forest that were clearly visible all over London following the crisis.

One of the nurses on the ward brought me a picture postcard of a Bristol Blenheim, the latest in RAF bombers.

'Daddy is a Squadron Leader', she said, 'and his squadron have just been equipped with new Blenheims.' With war so close at hand, I wonder what happened to Daddy?

The only detrimental thing about the HSC was the menu, an eternal round of mince or boiled chicken, while I could have lapped up an egg and chips.

It was becoming clear that I would not be out for Christmas and as December approached, plans were laid to ship me back to Stanmore whence I had come, a prospect I did not relish and a foreboding that was to be justified.

3

The Blight

The Royal National Orthopaedic Hospital at Stanmore in those days was a vast estate with wards scattered at intervals over the whole area and a ward discipline that would have done justice to a Borstal institution. Into this atmosphere I was literally dumped on to a very hard bed with a fracture board beneath the mattress and just left for days, no more were pressure points rubbed regularly or more than the barest of nursing care lavished on anyone. Beds and lockers had to be in line, all castor wheels turned under the bed, all counterpanes hanging true and level round the edges, all locker tops cleared and so on.

For the staff it was much the same, with nurses' uniforms having stiff starched collars with stud fastenings and stiff starched white cuffs that could be slipped off over the hands, placed one inside the other and stood on the nearest locker for the barest moment, before being whisked away by a small boy's hand and passed down the ward to an obscure hiding place. To leave the ward for any reason without those starched cuffs, a nurse could be put on a fizzer before some senior disciplinarian of the hospital.

The floors were polished with a bumper almost daily, a form of exercise to keep any man fit and healthy and the means of some simple entertainment for the patients, which is more than could be said for the ceremonial bedpan round which was enacted three times a day and you were required to conform. Any such call for relief outside ceremonial hours was officially frowned upon and with the beds in close proximity, there being no curtains or screen at any time, communal life was lived to the full, in a ward with forty eight

23

patients, between the ages of three and sixteen years. All were strictly orthopaedic patients who were not medically ill and so able to raise the customary exuberance of schoolboys despite their long stay prospects in hospital.

Come Christmas 1938, one of my long established desires was met. It actually snowed at Christmas time and lay deep and crisp and even over all the hospital grounds, but I was unable to set foot upon it and had never seen it lie so thickly before. Beautiful to look at, an enticement we could not meet and a great hazard to all those trudging visitors who came so loyally every Sunday afternoon for the two hour weekly visit.

Ward Sisters were fearsome and autocratic with an eagle eye for law and order, which they inflicted on nurses and patients alike. Many of the nurses were from South Wales and Ireland and all were pressed to the endless round of straightening beds, castors and lockers, as well as sweeping the ward floor every morning. Wards were built in pairs like semi–detached dwellings with a common duty room and the night shift would be one nurse to each ward and one junior to share between them. Read into this ninety-six patients to be wakened and washed every morning – the young children had to be washed and so did many of the older patients who were physically unable to perform this function – and it works out at thirty-two washes per nurse, plus a bottle round, hence the need for the 5 am start to the day.

Such was the world into which I had landed, a world that really had no time for anyone to be ill and so I suffered a great deal of unattended soreness on that hard bed, but worse was to come when the surgeon's round prescribed the current stock answer to polio – a plaster bed. To manufacture this device, you were trundled down the road to the plaster room where you were spread out on your face on the table, all your limbs were held more or less in the desired position and loads of hot wet plaster bandages smacked to and fro across your back until a thickness of plaster had been built up all over your body and legs right down to your toes. This morass would then be moulded to your personal contour, left to harden for a short time, then lifted off and stood aside while you were summarily washed down and returned to the ward. When the mould was set hard, it would be mounted on wooden blocks beneath, to raise the patient above the mattress those few vital inches to accommodate the utensil at each ceremonial round.

When your body and legs were spread out in this moulded plaster bed, you were theoretically the correct shape and free from deformity that can so easily set in with growing children who are paralysed, but it does not always work like that in practice and in my case, it all went terribly wrong. Unrubbed regularly by meths and powder since leaving Great Ormond Street and now laid on a thin blanket material straight into this hard plaster mould with none too smooth edges anywhere around, it was but a brief time before the inevitable happened and again I have to rely on the details subsequently given to me by another patient who became a great friend of mine – Alfie Gurney, nicknamed Fido!

It seems that I passed out and when someone noticed, I was turned out of the new plaster bed and there it was – a king size bed sore on the bottom vertebra. A great furore ensued and when I did come round, I was lying face down on that hard mattress and my bed was in the corner of the ward by the double doors to the bathroom and sluice. The length of time all this business occupied, I do not know, but what I do now know is that this was to be the real blight of my whole life.

Gradually my state of health improved, but I was kept lying flat on my face, so that dressings, inspections and ray lamps could all be applied in turn to my rear end. Back in the ward I found myself in the bed next to a bright fair haired lad of my own age and it was then that he related the foregoing details to me, for this was Fido.

4

The Eve of War

Alfie Gurney was probably the little flaxen-haired boy with the blue eyes that all the ladies love to spoil, but they never spoiled Alfie for their chance passed by when he contracted polio, which was not identified until he had been ill for some weeks and he was brought into Stanmore in a very poor state of deformity. He lay on the bed, propped up by a wickerwork backrest and his skinny near useless arms that had been crossed on his chest were now back on the pillow, with elbows permanently bent and the fingers rather curled, although they did retain some movement that could do little for him. His legs were equally skinny and both his feet were dropped, bent right down from the ankle in a way that made it painful to observe.

Apart from this, Alfie was very well and the greatest company for any long stay patient such as we all were on the ward. Always dreaming of when he grew up, we would air our increasing knowledge of orthopaedics by adding up all the operations that we thought would be necessary to get Alfie back to the right shape for future life – we carefully ignored the polio as if it were not there – a life that could be driving a lorry for Portland Cement, Blue Circle brand, as did his father back home in Dunstable.

Springtime was with us to herald that beautiful summer of 1939 and we all spent many hours out on the solarium, a concrete yard outside the ward where you could see out over the big green hill up to the dovecot at the top and the trees beyond, but our view of the girls in the adjacent ward who were also out on this concrete slab, was effectively blocked by a row of sight screens. I was still laid out on my face,

26

encouraged to get up on my elbows and feeling very well indeed by the time the ray lamps and other ponderings had healed over the bedsore, although this vertebra remained as a prominent protrusion on my back.

'We think it is sufficiently hardened now for you to be turned over on to your back,' they said.

So they turned me over and lo and behold, I could not lie flat on my back, which remained arched and when brought to the sitting position, my back still remained arched backwards and resisted all efforts to make it bend forwards in the normal manner. A severe kink backwards near the bottom of the spine had been brought about by months of lying on my face and being able to raise my shoulders and chest clear of the bed by resting on my elbows, a not uncomfortable posture at the time, bearing in mind the discomforts of the bedsore behind.

The blight that was to make the rest of my life far more difficult than it need have been was with me and they called it lordosis.

Sundry efforts were made to rectify the situation including a short session on one of the works of art of the acknowledged orthopaedic experts, the Fisher frame, a massive wooden structure that supported a gibbet from which the patient was suspended by a chin strap and loops under the arms and you were left in a sitting position with nothing to support your bottom. The theory was that this would stretch the spine, but the experiment on me did not last long and the existence of the lordosis was accepted as unadjustable.

Just before Easter a new patient walked into the ward, a small boy about ten years old with straight dark hair, an unhappy expression, and severe variation in the length of his legs. Ralph Herring spoke with a broad Yorkshire accent and was admitted as his parents had been convinced that modern medical science could do something to make good the six inches of bone and flesh that Ralph was lacking between the knee and hip on one leg, which made walking a great hazard for him. Ralph was studied and re-studied by the eminent men and others, and his bed was fitted up with a timber super-structure which provided two parallel beams, head to toe over the bed about four feet above the mattress.

When the great day came, Ralph was wheeled down the

road to the operating theatre which was in another block and his bed with the superstructure above, followed him. There was a very long time lag before the bed was wheeled back into the ward later in the day, indicating that a lot of work had been done and so it had, for slung from the cross beams was a hammock, in which lay the unconscious form of Ralph, with two boxes to support a pillow underneath his head. The rest of the set up was a little more complicated, as we eventually found that his body was shrouded in a short single spika – a plaster encasement from the waist, down over the hips and thence down to one knee on the fore-shortened side. Vertically through the plaster at the hip joint was a large steel pin which was embedded in the plaster fore and aft of the body, after passing through the flesh and bone of the leg. The knee itself was bent down with the foot on the bed and where the plaster ceased just above the knee, a steel hoop protruded from the plaster, out round the knee and back into the plaster, where it was very firmly embedded. A horizontal steel pin was inserted through the knee joint, much as the one at the hip and the protruding ends were coupled to a screw adjuster. We were told that the femur had been severed diagonally and the ends would grow together again despite the attentions of the houseman who came round each evening to give the screw adjuster a set number of turns, so increasing the distance between the two pins and theoretically lengthening the leg.

I awoke one night in that big ward with a high arched roof and was aware of someone singing. It was a choirboy voice with a Yorkshire accent singing lustily 'There is a green hill far away, beyond a city wall. . . '

When asked why he made all that noise in the night, he said words to the effect that he could not sleep, he did not want to cry, so he thought he had better sing. Such were the sufferings that could be intentionally inflicted on a small boy in 1939.

A few days later, Ralph was taken back to the operating theatre and all the elaborate paraphernalia was dismantled, for something had gone wrong. When he was brought back to the ward, his bed came up next to mine and when the time came round to dress his gaping wounds on his hip and buttock, where the pin had been extracted and similarly on his knee, there was time and cause for reflection on the ethics of the whole procedure. When the wounds were healed and Ralph was ready to go home, they made him a high boot to compensate for the seven and a half inches difference that then existed in that leg.

Visiting was for two hours on Sunday afternoons only and all the visitors were required to queue outside the main gate on Brockley Hill regardless of the weather until the hour of Two approached, when the gate keeper would open the ornamental iron gate and check all visiting cards before admitting anyone to the grounds of the hospital. Two cards only were issued to each patient and the only means of gaining admittance for any additional visitors was to pass the cards out through the railings to someone further back in the queue. Once inside the gate at two o'clock, it could be ten minutes hard walking through the grounds to reach the wards and this all came out of visiting hours, as the wards were cleared sharp at four o'clock. During an outbreak of diphtheria, on the ward, quarantine was declared and all the visitors lined up outside the windows to make apeing expressions at the boys inside, but somehow luck was on my side, as I was found to be naturally immune to diphtheria.

One of the highlights of the week was each Sunday morning, when a selection of Rover Scouts always came to run a Scout Troop on the ward. With 'Timber' Wood in charge, they were a lively crowd who ticked the weeks by for us with their never failing attendance and we all did our Morse code, our knots and many other things, but somehow we never got around to our Tracker Badges. They made Fido up to Patrol Leader, although we never actually patrolled anywhere and his interest in the Scout movement remained after he was sent home later that year to be pushed around the streets of Dunstable in a long wickerwork spinal carriage. Alfie was awarded a Cornwall Badge shortly before he succumbed to pneumonia in 1942 at the age of sixteen years. Alas, poor Fido.

A strange phenomenon of which I was unaware was going on behind those sight screens in the girls' ward next door. They did not allow Boy Scouts in there of course, for like us, the girls' ages ranged from three to sixteen years and they were left to the attention of the Girl Guides and Rangers on

Sunday mornings. Among the Guides attending was the elder sister of one of the patients on that ward, whom I had yet to meet.

Another bright spot was always provided by Mr Maud, a genial elderly gentleman who somehow managed to smuggle himself into the grounds and then into the children's wards, where he came up with sweets and comics, but this was all strictly frowned upon by ward sisters so that the whole exercise was a bit furtive. Those same ward sisters would always loom up on Sunday afternoons immediately visitors had departed and then make a systematic search of all lockers to confiscate any edible item they could find. The only safe solution to this was to stuff yourself silly while your visitors were there and to be violently sick when they had gone. This was not exactly a desirable solution, but it was proof against marauding sisters, which gave us some satisfaction.

The glorious hot summer was rolling by and we were spending all our days and some of our nights out on the solarium. During those days the beautiful green hill and the dovecote disappeared as a battery of new hutments were erected at great speed on the site. This formed a complete hospital in itself with theatre, X-ray and plaster rooms all complete, as an insurance against impending catastrophe and when that catastrophe was imminent there was a massive sifting of the patients, whence we all hoped to be sent home. Some of us were gratified, but the rest were moved to an old timber hut that served as a ward, near the main gate.

Those of us to be moved were wheeled in our beds out of the ward and down to the road where the beds were lined up in pairs, tied together side by side and then three pairs of beds were roped one behind the other to the back of a lorry which was driven at walking pace over the quarter mile to the old wooden ward, which had one side completely removed to satisfy the whim of the age that patients on the ward with tubercular joints needed fresh air, and good English fresh air at that! This was not a happy place for polio patients with wilting circulations, but those first few days of the war were far from a happy time for anyone. The row of beds nearest the open side had rubber draw sheets spread over the bottom of the beds to keep the bedclothes dry.

At about this time, the instrument makers came to start work on me and their first endeavour took a very long time to produce. Leg irons, known as callipers, provided a straight bar down each side of each leg and these were connected by deep steel bands behind each thigh and each calf and all tastefully upholstered in top quality leather covering. At the bottom of each leg, the side irons were sprung into a piece of gas barrel set in the heel of the boot and secured by massive tee straps. Round each knee was a complex strap and buckle collection with more buckles round the thighs and calves. The two leg irons were coupled up to another steel band round the pelvis and to be assembled into this was akin to harnessing a horse. This was the gadget of the age, built up bit by bit by the instrument maker as he worked and the odd innovations were invented as he went along, which tended to produce a Heath Robinson contraption that was decidedly uncomfortable to wear and very restrictive of the limb movement, particularly as the knees were permanently out straight. The cost in time and material must have been enormous, but when I was eventually harnessed up, I was still quite unable to sit up without holding on firmly with both hands, for the spinal deformity made me conspicuously pigeon chested and when sat up, my body would bulge forwards and fall flat on to my legs which were spread out in front of me.

The next little experiment was to make a plaster cast of my now weird shaped body, fill this plaster cast with more plaster to produce a solid full size model of me that could be knocked about. A great chunk of boot leather was then beaten round the model and moulded to the contours, trimmed off top and bottom, made to join down the front, lined with chamois leather, bound on the outside with steel strapping and then all built on to the existing pelvic band of the harness, making it sufficient for a shire horse. Incorporated in this structure was a mechanical locking device at each hip joint so that the body portion could be locked out in a straight line with the legs. This meant that the assembled harness complete with boots could be stood up on its own rather like a headless man. It also made it possible for me to be stood on my feet and to be put in a sitting position, although in that position I still tended to fall forwards and I was quite unable to sit back comfortably in a chair because of this tendency which is with me to this day, a source of great discomfort and inconvenience – and a blight on my whole life. A later modification added two big claw pieces to the body portion of the structure so that these would rest on the leg irons in the sitting position and so hold the body more or less upright in a chair, but the discomfort remained.

Ward Sister was a substantially built blonde, with an in-built hatred of little boys who fought mighty battles every morning with rubber bands and cigarette cards as pellets, that lay thick on the ward floor and gave rise to a great deal of vocal encouragement to the nurse to sweep up before Sister came on duty. A form of schooling was held on every ward, but the difficulties of teaching children of varying ages who were being constantly whipped away down the road for treatment or X-ray or plastering, was very great and no help was given to the benefits of tuition by small boys who pulled up the bedclothes and feigned sleep at crucial moments in the class.

The school mistress was a kindly soul who did her best under the circumstances and who was visited regularly by the headmistress, a petite lady of middle age, who wore a green overall coat and a green felt 'po' hat that we later came to associate with the WVS. It was this lady that had repeated cause to admonish the class over many weeks and all because of Joe.

Poor old Joe was a hospital employee and in this capacity, he was equipped with a wheelbarrow with which he visited the wards accompanied by his affliction – a large protruberance about the size of a Spanish onion which grew on one side of his nose and this unfortunate appendage would bounce up and down as he walked along, so causing the vision of that one eye to be severely restricted. The wooden hut had one small door along the back wall and my bed was next to that door, which had certain advantages, for every morning at the appointed hour, the door would open and there would be Joe with his wheelbarrow. As his foot fell on the floor of the ward, we were ready and a mighty chorus would ring forth,

'I'm coming, I'm coming and my head is bending low, I hear those gentle voices calling, Poor old Joe' and so on.

Joe would tramp down the ward breathing very foul and audible blasphemy about us, until he disappeared into the kitchen, when all would fall silent for a few brief moments while Joe raised a dustbin full of kitchen waste on to his shoulder and emerged from the kitchen to another chorus of 'Poor old Joe', as he carried the bin down the middle of the ward and out of the back door to his wheelbarrow.

Another strange thing about Joe, he always wore a green pork pie hat and when he came back into the doorway with the empty bin the chorus always changed to,

'Where did you get that hat, where did you get that tile? Isn't it a lovely one, quite the latest style' to which the response was more rude words about little boys.

Every morning Joe did four lengths of the ward on his dustbin round, every morning we did our ritual serenade and once a week Joe would complain to the headmistress about the boys on that ward. Being headmistress, she had to assert herself and she would arrive on the ward, raise her bottom on to one of the lockers to gain a little height, straighten the 'po' hat on her head and proceed with her set piece lecture.

'You are a naughty lot of little boys. That poor Mr So and So is only doing his job and you are to stop aggravating him like you have been doing.'

We all promised faithfully to behave, but by the time poor old Joe arrived next morning, our resolve had weakened and we all burst into our usual song. After some weeks we tired of this ritual and Joe was left comparatively unmolested in his work.

When Christmas came round again, the first Christmas of the war, we had a lot more snow and this was turned to our great entertainment by the Sunday morning visit of the Scouts who set to in the snow to wage a terrific battle with snowballs on the big yard outside the ward. This missing side of the building allowed us to be almost there in the battle, as near as could be imagined and it all served to warm our freezing bodies.

Another technique of warming was far less sought after, but nonetheless provided, after the evening TPRs (temperature, pulse and respiration) had been performed, there was always a check on your own performance with that delicate phrase 'Have you had a mark today?' Whatever your answer to that

question, the response was invariably unpleasant for they
seemed to have a knack of not actually believing your reply
and Sister's favourite recipe was for liquorice powder which
you could have thin enough to drink by the mugful or thick
enough to eat by the half mugful! There was seldom any
escape as administrative help was always at hand and the
results were pretty awful, remembering that we were all
permanently confined to bed and relief was expected to
coincide with the schedule of the bedpan rounds. The
warming part of the procedure was by Sister's special decree,
that you were down- or up- for an enema and we were
convinced that her dislike of you personally was reflected, as
it were, in the temperature of the water in that jug. Inner
cleanliness always came not only first, but most of the time.

The mugs in which the liquorice was served were quite
unique. They were bare metal pots holding about one third of
a pint each and a die cast handle was fixed to one side with
three rivets. As missiles they were excellent and could be
thrown at any fellow patient to whom you might take a
dislike and this process, together with normal domestic
handling, would slacken back the rivets and loosen the
handle so that when the mug was placed on your locker at
mealtimes and tea was brought round in a tall enamel jug to
be poured into the mugs, it became essential for you to gulp
that tea down forthwith before it all ran out of the rivet holes
in the side of the mug, all over your tiled locker top and down
to the floor.

Just such a missile was aimed one day at poor Gertrude, a
rather shy Irish nurse who was highly embarrassed by one of
the less gentlemanly patients who laid a mirror on the floor as
she made his bed and he then declared triumphantly to the
ward that Gertie was wearing pink underwear. The missile
incident concerned a little Irish patient with an ankle defect
and a short plaster up to one knee. At nine years of age he
was kept in a large cot which he used rather like a lion's cage
by marching round and round the railings and this he was
doing as poor Gertie arrived with the tea. She filled his mug
and handed it to him telling him to drink it.

'Shan't' he yelled, took the mug and hurled it and the tea
straight at Gertrude.

Tea splashed all down her white pinny and soaked through

to her pink undies and she stood there dripping on the floor. The commotion brought Staff to the scene and Gertrude was sent off duty, without her starched cuffs, to change into dry clean clothes, while Staff entered details of the offence in the duty book.

When Sister arrived on the ward later in the day, she studied the duty book, interviewed Staff, rolled up her sleeves, donned her elastic garters above her elbows and marched straight down the ward like Napoleon approaching Moscow. She slammed down the cot side, grasped Patrick firmly round the waist and carried him out of the back door by my bed to the green grass outside, where she laid him face down on the ground and administered corporal punishment with her own heavy hand. Undignified and unethical as it may have been, there was no doubt that the objective had been achieved swiftly and surely.

Visitors were still required to queue outside the gate and produce their visiting cards and on one of those days about this time, my mother was waiting in that queue when she got into conversation with another visitor, who it transpired, also lived in Wembley. Thus it was that I first met Roy, a fellow patient.

While all this was going on, I was having daily sessions in physiotherapy where I was trussed up in the whole harness, locked out straight and stood on my feet with a pair of crutches. Eventually I was able to strut up and down in a rather vague sort of way that did very little for me and the process of standing up and sitting down was almost impossible as I had to be locked in the straight position before pushing myself up out of the chair and had to lower myself into the chair in this rigid form.

Only after all this did anyone mention that a wheelchair might have its uses but the mention was somewhat half-hearted, since hospital tradition required you to be on your feet before discharge from the ward, so on your feet you had to be regardless of how useless the whole exercise might prove. The folding transit chair of today had not established itself in Britain at that time and the powers prescribed a wheelchair with backrest steering. There were lengthy harangues about paying for this vehicle and also about a modification for carrying my unbending knees, but eventually it arrived in May 1940. It was a weird contraption built entirely of flat strip steel sections and could be folded down like a pram, which achieved precisely nothing for it was exactly the same size folded down as unfolded, only a different shape. Two small bicycle wheels at the front each had a bicycle chain running up vertically to a hand crank, one for each hand and the backrest of the seat was fixed to a central pivot so that by leaning left or right you could turn the single rear wheel in the desired direction of travel. This was moderately successful but I still had to strap my sagging body to the backrest to remain in position in the chair.

With this vehicle I was allowed out on very brief sorties from the ward which gave me a limited view of the world outside for the first time in nearly two years. No-one brought newspapers and there was no radio on the ward, so the affairs of the world were effectively isolated from us. We knew there was a war on, but it made little difference to us in the hospital, until one day soon after getting the chair, I propelled myself round the corner to the Main Gate of the hospital in time to witness a sight that made me think. The gate porter opened both wrought iron gates and a Green Line coach drove slowly into the entrance, followed by a whole convoy of Green Line coaches, all of which had been withdrawn from their regular pre–war duties in and around London and been converted into large ambulances. Hardly two vehicles in the convoy were alike but each was loaded with wounded men, many on stretchers in tiers inside the coaches and other walking wounded standing in the open doorways in the bright May sunshine as the convoy wound its way slowly through the lanes of the hospital grounds to fill those new hospital hutments that had been built the year before. The war was quite suddenly a reality to me.

5

Home and Away

Soon after this I was told that I was being discharged and I, together with the wheelchair was eventually collected by the Wembley Borough Council ambulance that day in early June 1940 when Italy declared war on Great Britain. Reaching home, I was carried inside by the ambulance men and they sat me back in the Windsor armchair with the assurance that I would be alright there. This seemed to be the general view of so many people then and still that of a few people today. If you are disabled you are out of the normal run of life and you should sit back and not strain yourself but economic necessity does not come within their vision when they offer this advice.

It was nice to be home after nearly two years in hospital and the ritual of being wheeled out in the wheelchair began and people called to visit and offer pastimes, usually books and magazines. Time did pass quite quickly with the only real problems arising from breakages of the harness which had to be taken back to Stanmore for repair. Among the literature that rolled up for study was the Railway Magazine and from this I learned a great deal more about my observations from the back windows of the house and about the faraway places in the Highlands that sounded so lovely in the narrative of the articles. Oban, Fort William and Mallaig were places to dream about at the end of long straggling railway lines and I concocted my own visions of what they were really like but gave not a thought to ever seeing them.

The war seemed to be getting blacker and blacker. We listened every night to the nine o'clock news and to all the fiery broadcasts by Churchill, again without realising the gravity and historical significance of spoken words. Nights were spent in the Anderson shelter and even the cat knew when to take cover. Not that very much happened in Wembley, but during the height of the blitz, the red night sky over East London was clearly visible from the garden. My first Christmas at home was very much under these conditions, the months were rolling by and thoughts were being given to my interrupted education, but it did not get far beyond the thought stage until the 'Week's Good Cause' appeal was made by Derek McCulloch for the Training College for the Disabled at Leatherhead, of which we had never heard. I wrote for details, which looked as though they might offer me something useful and this was put to the Education Department in Middlesex with a reminder that I had been unable to take up the eleven plus place that I had won in 1938.

In the summer of 1941, I had a brief stay on the ward in Stanmore while the harness was amended and repaired as breakages were a constant source of discomfort to me. During that stay I met a certain practical joker whose exploits were rather too extreme for laughter. Such an occasion was when a less than bright patient was sitting on a bed pan in full view of the whole ward and along comes the wag, who pushes a piece of newspaper down the tubular handle of the pan and sets fire to it. The less than bright patient was able to raise himself high off the pan in mid action while the flames momentarily licked round his bottom in sterilising fashion. A very dangerous and stupid thing to do and how fortunate that no real harm came to anyone. On another occasion I myself was the victim of his hilarity. Having been placed in the ward bath and left to soak, a hand that I recognised came through the open window and deposited something upon my head, which I instinctively raised a wet hand to remove. The damp of my hand had the effect of congealing the deposit in my hair into an evil smelling mass of green flakes of enema soap.

Eventually the Education Committee agreed to place me at Leatherhead and in February 1942, I was on my way into the Surrey countryside.

Leatherhead Court was a country mansion of no great age with a main door in the centre of the long front facade with steps to the approach. Inside was a large banqueting hall with a grand staircase leading up to a balcony on three sides of the hall. Behind these grand appointments was a large untidy courtyard with the buildings flanking both sides, where an archway led out into the grounds. Behind all this again came the stable blocks made up into workshops to teach gas welding to those sitting down, electric arc welding for the one armed, a full range of machine tools, a bench fitters' class where the prime test was to file a one inch cube from solid steel to a fine tolerance and dead square all ways round. Also for the one armed was paint spraying and the rest was made up of the Handyman section, a bit of pen pushing and a Drawing Office.

Accommodation was in rooms upstairs and in the side wing of the main building, food on a meagre scale was taken in the main hall and recreation was catered for by a billiard table and a branch of the County Library.

After surveying the options open to me, I elected to enter the Drawing Office where it took nearly three months to get away from printing alphabets and numerals before attempting to draw a sausage. Not that drawing sausages was even attempted, the customary text book instruction was worked through very thoroughly before being allowed to dismember spray guns, oxy-acetylene torches and the like and to draw every detail for minute inspection.

Academic work was done in a separate classroom with a stout elderly gentleman who might well have stepped out of Greyfriars except that his approach to mathematics was somewhat unorthodox. Since none of his class were able to act as monitors and he himself carried far too much weight to take any unnecessary steps, he developed the technique of sitting at his desk in front of the class and throwing the textbooks to each pupil as if he was playing hoop-la. It was not very good for the books but it did waste some time retrieving them from the floor when you were unable or unwilling to catch them in full flight. Why this schoolmasterly figure was known as Sabu I could never imagine for he resembled the elephant rather than the boy. When Sabu eventually sank into his chair never to rise again a new schoolmaster arrived full of bristle and vim; Major Something or Other, they said he was and by gad, Sir, what a lad, sir! On sunny summer afternoons he always trailed the class out of the schoolroom into the grounds, where we all sat around the park benches to digest algebra and trigonometry, or at least, that was the idea. Once launched on trigonometry, the odd tactfully placed question would launch this ex-Sandhurst man into a lengthy dissertation on the technicalities of range finding for artillery or navigation by the stars – all fascinating stuff, but of little value to our educational programme but nonetheless a very pleasant way to pass an afternoon on a bench in the gardens. The other great distraction from work was the weekly session of making copies of your drawings by the very basic vintage methods of blue printing in a large frame exposed to the sunlight for an arguable length of time, followed by washing the prints under the yard tap and hanging them out like the weekly washing to dry.

On the odd occasions that distinguished visitors were conducted round the workshops and offices, it was desirable to develop the technique of drawing, erasing and re-drawing the same line over and over again at snail's pace, in the hope that you would convey the impression of skill and accuracy. This also ensured that you did not make an extra error with a critical eye watching over you.

Accommodation was hardly luxurious and Room 8 was equipped with eight beds, eight lockers, mostly old chests of drawers, a large wardrobe and two fire places which left room to ride round in my Richards wheelchair. Wartime economy was impressed upon us by our over zealous management when they reduced the wattage of the light bulbs all round the dormitories and Room 8 with a very high ceiling and fitted out as described, was awarded a single fifteen watt bulb on a short flex. Twinkle, twinkle, little star, how we wonder where we are!

Constant companions in all the rooms were the mice who rummaged through the lockers for any edible morsel that we were unwise enough to leave there. One of the few extras in our room was Joe's gramophone with a pile of elderly records which we played with monotonous regularity and the most stirring of these was the National Emblem March, which usually brought a Geordie voice from the next room to sing the sweet refrain 'Have you ever caught your finger in a mousetrap?' The other monotonous regularity was the ex-barrack square voice from the garden calling the housey-

housey numbers to the halfpenny gamblers around him.

Gambling in halfpennies was what most of us were reduced to by the meagre standards of everything that could keep body and soul together. If you were installed in the College by the Ministry of Labour you could draw a full guinea a week, but if you were there by courtesy of a County Education Authority, you had to assemble on Fridays at the billiard table and the deputy superintendent would open his little bag and shoot the silver only out on the table, then read down his list of names and push the appropriate coinage across the table towards you. The monetary value of the coinage depended on the Local Authority responsible for your presence and the best offer was five shillings for a few, with half a crown for the most and for the remaining unfortunates including Joe and myself, there was one shilling to come. This was the 'College Bob' which was paid to every trainee to ensure that none were entirely without.

Meagre standards of catering were also a feature of the establishment based on that good old stand–by 'There's a war on'. In reality the housekeeper married the one-legged cook and they would depart at weekends with more than a weekend bag and all conveyed in the town taxi-cab, a large fawn Standard saloon from the early nineteen thirties. After breakfast it was customary for all those able to rush up to the serving table to be given a small helping of dripping from the bacon pan, to be spread on the bread available at the table and all necessary to maintain the strength of a working man. At one stage, there was an inexhaustable supply of kippers which were very tasty, but did become a little wearing when applied like medicine in regular doses. The most intriguing part of the kipper glut was the clearing of the plates, when the residue was tipped into the dustbins outside to remain therein until the kitchen waste contractor called each week, by which time the lids could be seen to rise and fall in constant rhythm of their own volition and the affluvia was unbearable.

Domestic rations at that time included a large helping of cheese, from which my mother was able to keep me well stocked up together with a plentiful supply of dates and very hard biscuits which resembled dog biscuits. These three items alone served to keep myself and my Geordie friend Bill from the bitterest pangs of hunger and were known to us as 'stand-by'.

Following lunch one day, there was considerable disquiet about the food and the trainees all gathered in the courtyard to moan to one another, when some loud mouth climbed on a chair and started yelling that we were not going back to work until we had had a decent lunch. This produced three cheers on all sides and also produced the Superintendent, who was a less than inspiring officer retired from the RAF. This limp figure was in a state of near panic by the strike of trainees and well he might have been, for this very afternoon, the Governing Committee were due to make their annual patronising visit to survey the good works being done at the College and be carefully steered away from the seamier details of our existence. The Committee, headed by Dame Georgina, a daughter of the famous General Buller of Boer War fame, could have been expected to throw a fit had they witnessed the demonstration in the courtyard, but as it was, it was the Group Captain who nearly threw the fit with his beggings and pleadings and promises of a better tomorrow for all of us undernourished trainees. The Superintendent's theatricals even touched the heart of the agitator standing on the chair and so we all trailed back to the workshops behind the building just as the Committee arrived in the driveway, so allowing the poor Group Captain to stabilise his pulse rate.

The effects of wartime thinking were reflected in the change of title of the establishment which had been working for years as the Cripples Training College, when· it came under the patronage of the Queen and was christened the Queen Elizabeth Training College for the Disabled. This was doubtless brought about by the increasing number of discharged service men then coming into the College for training for civilian employment. Many of these men were ambulatory and a petition was then sent to the Queen, which pressurised London Transport into providing a Saturday afternoon bus from the College into the town of Leatherhead two miles away. This two miles was a very long trundle in the Richards wheelchair particularly when you were on your own and the gradients of the town were formidable for this sort of vehicle. The more affluent trainees were able to club together for a taxi and once in the town your accumulated 'college bobs' would get you into the Crescent Cinema – now the Sybil Thorndyke Theatre – and up the High Street to the Bluebird Café where we always had cheese on toast, a great luxury to us, before setting out on the two mile lone trek back to the college.

It was on one of these return trips that I could have met my Waterloo, as the Canadian Army Post Office were set up in a field just on the edge of the town and with darkness falling, I pedalled straight into the deep mud at the entrance to the camp and there stuck fast. I had visions of the jeeps and trucks roaring up the lane and into the camp at their usual breakneck speed, but fortunately nothing happened and after a lengthy wait, a passerby managed to extract me from the mire in the middle of the camp entrance and I made my way home caked in mud.

On another day I trundled out into the lane outside Leatherhead Court and was somewhat alarmed to hear the screech of a strident steady–note siren that I knew was not the customary warning of an air raid. The tone grew louder and was obviously approaching from somewhere, but I knew not where, as I backed the chair up into the hedge to become as inconspicuous as possible, lest the threatened invasion had begun and was heading my way.

The hedge would provide little protection, but it was my first thought to become an ostrich and bury my head in the sand, which was a physical impossibility for me and anyway, there was no sand, only the green lush fields of Surrey all around me.

The sound grew nearer and more raucous and eventually an army convoy roared round the corner from the Cobham direction – half a dozen army staff cars, Humber Snipes with razor edge bodies, the first of which carried the blaring siren that screamed incessantly and they raced towards Leather-head at very high speed, carrying I know not whom to I know not where, but obviously on an urgent mission.

The Richards wheelchair had small propelling wheels and a top speed little more than walking pace, but Joe had a larger and much older version of this machine with twenty six inch wheels and a greater turn of speed. So it was that I borrowed Joe's chair one fateful Sunday afternoon and en route to Fetcham disaster struck. I had been accustomed to propelling the Richards with one hand and pressing the other hand on the opposite chain case to control the backrest steering. Just such a manoeuvre I thoughtlessly tried on Joe's machine that afternoon forgetting that somewhere in its history, someone had removed the protective chain cases, leaving the bicycle chains and sprockets exposed before your very hands. The process was swift and painless, but the net end result was the amputation of the little finger of my left hand down to the second knuckle, an operation performed in Leatherhead Cottage Hospital a few days later.

The occasional journeys home were from Leatherhead Station to Waterloo in the Electric Multiple Units then in use. These were elderly ex-steam stock converted to electric traction and fitted up with strange vee-fronted driving cabs. To be loaded wheelchair and all into the guard's van was usual and the guard would back you up against a cross partition and then stack all the ARP sandbags round the chair wheels, an operation made necessary by the very violent take-up and braking of these trains.

The months at the college ticked by and the basic course was completed with a few re-runs of some of the items, but there seemed no great efforts being made to place me in employment until the autumn of 1943 when I visited the Youth Employment Office at the local authority in Wembley, where I was interviewed by a young lady who promised to get me a job – a tall order in those days, but the chances were improved by the Act of Parliament then recently introduced by Ernest Bevin as Minister of Labour and National Service, which required employers of more than twenty people to accept three per cent of their payroll from the new disabled persons' register.

Since my days at Leatherhead, the establishment has become the Queen Elizabeth Foundation for the Disabled and absorbed the old Ronson Industries factory in Oaklawn Road and Dorincourt became a sheltered workshop that eventually took in printing as well as a proliferation of ceramics.

It was to see the printing processes with a view to having the *Magic Carpet,* which came much later in my life, produced at Queen Elizabeth's, that I visited Leatherhead in 1982 for a conducted tour of the entire establishment including the room where we slept and the old stable or cowshed that served as a Drawing Office. The tour was conducted by the gentleman to whom I had previously submitted a copy of the chapter from this epistle relating to my days as a trainee in 1942, all in response to their request for such reminiscences of the forties and fifties to build up their archives.

Uncomplimentary as my story would read, all concerned at QE seemed highly delighted with the tale and as we progressed from workshop to workshop in 1982, my guide would announce triumphantly 'This gentleman was here forty years ago!' The response was such that I felt like Methusala and was stared at accordingly.

On 13 December 1943, I started work in a steel office furniture factory in the Exhibition Grounds in Wembley although much of the work there at that time was anything but furniture.

The factory was a seething mass of people with crowds of women all working diligently away in an atmosphere of tension that caught the imagination as you entered the building. The cry was production, the roof lights were blacked out and the plant was run round the clock. During daylight hours 'the little man' was in charge and he kept the pot boiling with his effervescence and ability to be everywhere at once as the sole management on site.

Ammo boxes, shelving, lightweight ships' furniture, massive cabinets for radar or radio equipment and ammunition tracks for bombers were all in production here. These tracks were made of stainless steel, sheared and formed in channel section and assembly was by zintex brackets which held two channels apart as a track for the passage of belts of bullets, first for .303 and later .5 machine guns.

The tracks were formed on the Cerrobend process that involved filling each channel with a low melting point metal to make it into a solid bar, whence it could be curved up, down, right or left as required for assembly and the whole would come up as a complete scenic railway to be mounted by the brackets into the fuselage of the bomber.

Complete kits for Lancasters went by lorry to A V Roe in Manchester and the Halifax tracks were sent to Chiswick bus works of London Transport from where the fuselages were transported to Leavesden airfield for final assembly and flying off.

A rather crude structure in the factory formed a canteen from out of which came an ample supply of good food with a relay system for lunches, but the canteen came into its own at Christmastime not so much for the basic celebrations, but for the residue of the Pig Club.

Undeveloped land at the back of the factory was used for a few allotments and the company Pig Club presided over by George Branch as chief pigman. George was really the steel stores keeper and goods inwards man, supervising the endless stream of ancient Thorneycrofts from the GWR delivering steel sheets from the railway yard at Park Royal. In his other hat he would push his large barrow round the local factories collecting the waste food bins for his great big stew pot that boiled everything to pulp. Bins from the other factory at Victoria came every day in the regular LNER mechanical horse that was contracted to ply between the two factories of the company. George would always voice his wrath about canteen women who put tea leaves in the bins for apparently pigs do not appreciate these as a delicacy.

Come Christmas, the fat porkers would be loaded into the company lorry for shipment to the Wall's meat pie factory at Acton where the unfortunate beasts would be stood on a steel plate, have ear phones applied and at the press of a button would heel over, to be dragged away, split open, degutted and the half carcasses thrown back on the van. This service was provided by Wall's without charge just to obtain the intestines that would be mangled into the next pork pie.

The company had a series of nicknames for many of the people there and George with his sparsely populated head of hair was known as Gooseberry. Another unfortunate who was chargehand of the girls working the spot welders, was blessed with an over generous nose and duly nicknamed 'Honky'. A certain naive young lady in his charge did one day address him as 'Mr Honk' and there was an embarrassed silence.

The atmosphere and urgency of war time production was never again attained in the Art Metal factory which goes a long way to explain the decline in Britain at the time of writing.

Coming to eighteen years of age in 1944 and well clear of conscription by my disability, I nonetheless registered on the appointed day and the elderly clerk on duty completed the form by writing 'cripple' across the paper. He then handed me a leaflet telling me I had 'better have one of these as everyone else had one'. I took it home, ready it carefully and was sorely tempted to fill it in and post it, thus indicating my willingness to become a Bevin Boy, the option open to conscripts to serve in the coal mines instead of the fighting services.

Travel was still with the Richards and the whole thing was getting rather weak at all its myriad rivetted joints and well worn on its not uncomplicated bearings, but it managed to drag on until the end of the war when I bought a Trilox lever propelled tricycle with twin chain two speed drive under the seat and a few peculiar details of construction such as ordinary caliper brakes acting on knucklesided wheelrims which were decidedly ineffective when free wheeling. This was rectified by fitting a new front wheel with a drum brake so that downhill stretches could be attempted with some degree of safety.

With the Trilox it was possible to cover more ground and one or two excursions were undertaken with my father marching along beside. He had always been a great walker and on the first of these jaunts we set out for Hampstead Heath and the familiar surroundings of Spaniards Road and then down into the Vale and up on to Parliament Hill, a great vantage point overlooking London Town. This was a fair step for a day's walk and I repeatedly tried to persuade him to let me trundle on for a mile or two while he took a bus or train to our next meeting point, but it was clearly evident that he was intent on walking with me all the way there and back.

On our greatest marathon, we met an astonished neighbour in Kilburn High Road and I often wondered what that neighbour would have thought had he known that we did the length of the Edgware Road, turned along Marylebone Road and onward to Kings Cross, Grays Inn Road, Holborn and eventually to St Paul's. Not that there was any access to the cathedral for me but the things to be seen at walking pace are seldom noticed from a motor car. It was a long day and a tiring one especially for my father then in his early fifties, but a day I remember and one that I appreciated for the effort involved.

It was during this period of inactive leisure time that I took out the paint box I had in my school days and put this together with a similar box of great vintage and launched myself into the production of a series of large watercolour paintings of locomotives and trains. The quality was never brilliant but I did derive great satisfaction from these efforts and they filled my long evenings at home, listening to the radio. Each was a scaled up version of a postcard or photograph of some kind and often featured the scenes I had witnessed on the Metropolitan in days gone by.

Seeking a further improvement in my transport, I saved hard to buy a three speed Carter lever propelled chair, but this also had its disadvantages, as the trail on the front forks was insufficient to get the weight behind the front wheel and so maintain a straight course when in motion. This tendency to erratic steering soon led me to sell this machine and return to the Trilox where the back axle was no longer very true, which caused both back wheels to wobble alarmingly, but before the Carter was disposed of, it was put to use by Cyril Porter who struggled on to the train at Wimbledon Park and came to Wembley on Cup Final days just to boast to the neighbours that he was 'going to Wembley'. After lunch we set off in the two hand propelled trikes to join the crowd outside the stadium to see Prince Philip and Princess Margaret arrive and to hear that two supporters in motor tricycles had come from Blackpool with tickets and were refused entry to the stadium with the trikes. They ended up in the TV monitor van to watch the match from outside the walls. Nearly thirty years later the same inflexible attitude remained at Wembley Stadium.

A strange sequence of events that could be thought of as uncanny, concerned the bungalow that stood in Barnhill Road, just three doors from our own house. Built in two thirds of an acre of land, it was occupied by a railway guard from the Metropolitan and his wife, a kindly soul who befriended my mother just after the traumatic days of August 1938 and often came to visit me in Great Ormond Street Hospital with her.

In the summer before the war, we learned that the bungalow was owned by this lady's mother who was of a less than amenable nature, which attitude showed clearly when she sold the bungalow and the residents had to move out. It was fortunate that a railway cottage was available in Neasden Village and they were thus able to live there, meanwhile the new owner had a lot of building and decorating work done before his planned arrival in Barnhill Road.

Part one of this strange story then happened, for on the eve of moving in, the new owner suddenly died and the property was eventually put up for sale again. War was very near and eventually the sale was agreed and a lady with two little boys moved in and we learned that their father was in the Merchant Navy and away at sea, a truly perilous occupation for any man in 1940.

The bad news of the early months of war at sea came in regularly on the radio and in the newspapers and when the day came that we met Mrs Ball and her two little lads along the road, she shed a few tears. A telegram had come that morning to say that her husband had gone down on the *Jarvis Bay*, in one of the most epic acts of bravery performed at sea in those days.

The bungalow was again for sale and as time rolled by, the next new owners arrived and much in evidence was a lady with a raucous voice and dyed ginger hair. She was of a family of street traders and at dawn each morning a lorry would arrive from Covent Garden and unload a young mountain of fruit and veg to be followed shortly afterwards by a pony and cart. The driver would go indoors for breakfast leaving the pony to trail the cart all over the garden and eat his way through every growing thing there before loading up and away to the stall in some odd spot.

Meanwhile the ginger lady's husband was involved in a road transport business and would sometimes park a 30 cwt Commer van in the driveway of the bungalow and that is where part three of this story began. In 1944 that van and its driver were 'somewhere in Cambridgeshire' when an American fighter plane crash landed right on top of the van killing the driver, the third owner of that bungalow to die in five years.

With the war over, the railway guard who originally lived there, quite suddenly developed a terminal illness and that uncanny sequence of events in the history of that bungalow was over.

6

The Open Road

It was early in 1948 that a copy of the Infantile Paralysis Fellowship Bulletin arrived and included a slip of paper announcing the formation of the Invalid Tricycle Association. This sounded more interesting, so I sent my five shillings subscription and back came a receipt from Robert Lee, the Founder Secretary, with a letter from O A Denly, the Chairman, upon whose exploits the ITA had been conceived.

It transpired that in 1947 Mr Denly had been all the way across Europe to Switzerland in his Argson de Luxe Motor tricycle with a folding wheelchair strapped on to the side and upon his return to England he was interviewed on BBC Radio to relate his story of the journey and this was followed by a two page feature in the magazine *Motor Cycling*. Together these items produced enough correspondence and interest to found the Invalid Tricycle Association with a small Management Committee, all of whom were Invalid Tricycle drivers.

The basic rule of the ITA was that only disabled people could become full members, that no committee could include more than two able-bodied Associate members and only full members would be allowed to vote at any meeting. This forced the issue of disabled people doing a great deal more than most of them ever imagined they could achieve and my five shillings did just that for me.

At this time I was still hand-propelling the Trilox and looking wistfully at motor tricycles, when the first copy of the ITA magazine *The Magic Carpet* arrived, bearing stories of exploits with trikes and the proclamation of a National Rally at the army camp in Richmond Park in August 1948.

In early June 1948, Cyril and I were both on the road with new Argson 'Victory' motor tricycles, just one month before the National Health Service came into being. The acquisition of this tricycle was probably the greatest step forward in my life up to then, for despite the primitive structure of the vehicle, its ability to cover the ground and clock up the miles was undoubted.

A tubular steel frame, with rigidly mounted back wheels, a sprung front wheel, a bucket seat on tiny coil springs in tension, so that should they fail you would drop straight through to the road. A rear mounted two stroke engine of 147 cc with fan cooler built in was coupled to a two speed gearbox driving the lefthand wheel. Propelling levers for manual forward and reverse were coupled to the right hand wheel with a dog clutch and steering was by a stirrup on the right hand propelling lever.

The process of learning to drive was a combination of experience of propelling the Trilox with swotting and practising the procedures in the instruction manual of the Argson. The vehicles were similar in that they both had propelling levers, but the Argson had the additional strenuous exercise of starting the engine with a hand lever attached to the kick start of the gearbox and many a pint of sweat was to be generated on this function. It was usually easier to take the huge 18mm sparking plug out of the cylinder head, give it a brisk polish, replace it, offer a brief prayer and then lay on the starting handle again!

With 'L' plates up and the initial driving practice complete, Cyril drove over from Wimbledon and we set out 'for the country' – not that we had the least idea where the countryside was from Wembley Park, but I did have recollections of a train journey from Wembley Park to Chorleywood, so we set out to follow the railway line in that direction. This brought us crossing and re-crossing the line at almost every bridge, a protracted means of progress but a very interesting one as it brought us on to many minor roads in the area. It took all afternoon to reach Pinner and there we saw another trike with a lady driver, so we gave chase, but a distant sight is all we ever had, as she must have lived locally and disappeared into her own backyard. This was one of many short trips out that we did at weekends, sometimes from Wembley and at others from Wimbledon, but when the company holiday came round, we planned more adventurous journeys, the first of which was on the Tuesday when I announced at home that I was going to Wimbledon and then 'out for a ride'. In his younger days, Cyril had been a keen cyclist, the 'Brighton before breakfast' brigade, so we set out to relive the road to Brighton on a glorious long hot summer day, with the open road entirely to ourselves as we were among the few privileged people to have a good supply of petrol coupons, for Pool Petrol at 2/1½d a gallon – plus a little oil for the two-stroke.

How marvellous it all was, as Sutton and Reigate rolled by, then we crossed into Sussex down the A23 over the Downs into Brighton town, past the Pavilion and we turned on to the road above Madeira Drive with miles of bright blue sea spread out before us. A sight I had never before seen and one that we sat back to enjoy before we supped our sandwiches and talked of the journey home. The miles did seem rather endless, as they often do on a strange road, but we arrived back in London without any mechanical bother. I left Cyril in Wimbledon and headed for Putney Bridge and Hammersmith en route home, where I announced that we had been to the seaside for the day, to which the response was a stunned silence of disbelief, so I did not breathe a word about our next journey planned for Thursday.

On that morning I set out along the Bath Road and met Cyril at Taplow station. With more sunshine overhead we were off westwards along the Floral Mile through the avenue of tall popular trees that lined the main road, over Sonning Bridge and into Reading where I decided on the only road known to me from childhood. The main road past the Brooke Bond and Huntley and Palmer factories was followed for miles until we reached Tilehurst with still no sign of Prospect Park, so a few enquiries took us over the hill and back on to the Bath Road towards Theale where we studied the map for the turning to Aldermaston village. On past the derelict airfield and there was Baughust, a straggling village just over the border in Hampshire to where Ernie Evans had recently retired. It took a good deal of research to find his new home at Stone Lodge but at last we arrived and drove in side by side through the five barred gate and parked at the front door. Cyril climbed out of his trike and was walking slowly round the house when I heard his very polite tones say 'Good afternoon, sir, I've brought someone to see you.'

They both walked back towards the front door and the customary stolid Evans manner left Ernie the moment he saw me. He rang back to the kitchen calling to my Aunt Lil and what a wonderful welcome we both had, for it was ten years since I last visited his home and this visit was quite a surprise, but not the least bother, as two pairs of double doors were flung open and I propelled the trike straight into the lounge and up to the tea table.

The peace and solitude of Baughurst was wonderful, the only sounds were the birds, the occasional cow or tractor and the twice a day bus from Basingstoke passing the door. We headed home via Basingstoke and the A30 and I left Cyril somewhere after Staines to pursue his way back to SW19. When I arrived in Wembley and said we had had tea in Baughurst, there was another stunned silence, but it soon wore off and stories of the journey followed.

In August the Rally at Richmond Park drew two hundred tricycles from all over the country and most daily papers carried reports and some pictures of the egg and spoon races and other similar events. It was an unforgettable day, making many acquaintances, some of whom were later to become friends and even relations of mine. This was also the day and the place where my mother and her three sisters were last photographed together, although we knew none of this at the time.

The other great event of 1948 brought the Olympic Games to Wembley with immense reconstruction work in the Exhibition grounds and at Wembley Park station, prior to the ceremonial opening of the Games. The only visible signs outside the walls of the stadium were the endless crowds of people but this all changed with the marathon.

The full field left Wembley that day and during the afternoon they were trailing home from their jaunt to St Albans in a very thin and weary stream and as the very last man staggered over the hill by Wembley Town Hall, there right on his heels was a very large ambulance already loaded with stricken athletes and right at hand to collect another.

7

The Invitation

Soon after Christmas 1948 I received a circular with a 1d stamp on it from a Mr Donald Booth, a member of the ITA who lived in Wealdstone informing me that he was hoping to set up a local group of the Association in the area. I replied to this letter offering my support to any group he might be able to form, without realising that I was about to become involved in the work of a lifetime. Another circular arrived from Mr Booth and this invited me to a meeting at Uxbridge, in the works canteen of the Bell Punch Company, where one of our members was employed.

Cyril arrived in Wembley on that Saturday morning and after lunch we set out for Uxbridge and in the little side streets off the High Street we crossed a hump backed canal bridge, turned on to the tow path and there were the doors of the canteen opening almost on to the canal bank. Outside were parked a selection of tricycles all of varying manufacture and design, and inside the canteen much the same could be said of their drivers who were sitting there in not so neat lines, mostly on canteen chairs, but one or two still in their trikes and at a top table there were three gentlemen and one lady. Everyone was looking just a little self-conscious; well almost everyone!

There were thirty three people at that meeting and my immediate companion was the only person known to me then, but over the coming months, I was to learn a lot about most of the people present that afternoon, those people who would become involved in that lifetime of activity and achievement.

At the centre of the table sat a handsome well-groomed

54

young man with a neat Clark Gable moustache who introduced himself as Don Booth, the instigator of our meeting at Bell Punch. Don had been discharged from the RAF having developed multiple sclerosis, a form of disability that I had not previously seen and a condition that affected his stability on his feet and was alleged to be progressive, but was clearly proving no great hindrance to his ability to get both the miles and the speed out of his tricycle. This was an 'Invacar' with a little Villiers 125 cc three speed unit mounted in front of the offside back wheel and a comfortable bucket seat slung between the back wheels, rather like a sidecar outfit being driven from the sidecar. It was much larger than my own machine and was among the first of its kind to use tiller bar steering with depression braking.

Sitting beside Don at the table was an older man of small stature with thinning sandy hair, a moustache, gold rimmed spectacles and a worried look, brought on when Don introduced him as Bob Laughlin, an employee of the Bell Punch Company who had acquired the hall for our meeting and should therefore be honoured as chairman for the afternoon, a task for which he was obviously ill prepared. Bob was living in lodgings in Uxbridge and was the owner of another 'Invacar'. His disability was a selection of congenital malformations that allowed him to walk short distances with the aid of a walking stick.

The young lady was a friend of Don's and an obvious admirer, although she said nothing throughout the entire meeting. She had driven a rather splendid looking Deluxe Argson from Bushey and she walked about on crutches at a slow pace as a result of a pre-war epidemic of poliomylitis. Her name was Gwen Taylor and she had been a patient in Stanmore Orthopaedic Hospital in the times previously recalled and she had an elder sister who had helped to run the Guide Company on that ward in those days.

Next to Miss Taylor sat a well built jovial looking man in his mid thirties who paid great attention to his pipe as all pipe smokers seem to do. Reg Bolton had some form of paralysis of the legs and always struggled round on a very flimsy pair of crutches which now stood behind his chair. A married man with a mundane clerical job in a Greenford factory, his whole life was wrapped up in his well equipped workshop at home from which he was able to produce some very high quality engineering work to private order. Reg owned two Argson tricycles as a guarantee of mobility and both were powerful versions with 197 cc Villiers engines of cast iron pot and piston vintage.

Sitting near the front of the meeting was an elderly and prosperous looking gentleman who really belonged to the bowler hat and brolly brigade, but had succumbed to the painful effects of extensive arthritis. This was Mr Marsland, or Dave to his friends, who became fewer as we got to know him, or rather to know his trike. This was an extraordinary machine made by Barrett in Bath. The conventional invalid carriage layout was retained and the seat had plywood sides sweeping up to shoulder level and downwards again to the rear where a button down canvas cover obscured the works. Above the seat at shoulder level was the mounting for a large black pram hood that could be raised above the driver's head to form a sort of air scoop or parachute brake and the front corners of the hood had long straps attached which came down to the front corners of the seat. A stem from the front forks carried the handlebars and fixed on the handlebars was a perspex windscreen that would swing from side to side with the steering, thus vaguely protecting the driver from the elements while his legs were covered with a canvas apron. Springs were fitted between the seat and the frame and when in action with a heavyweight driver aboard, the effect was for the frame and the rear wheels to bounce up and down under the seat as he progressed over the imperfections of the roadway. This machine was once described as a 'Howdah' on wheels with Dave Marsland making a very realistic Rajah in an Afrika Corps hat.

Thirty three disabled people attended this meeting and all except one came by trike and although many of them did not enter the discussion at all, there had to be one man who had more to say than all the others put together and it is strange that he should be one of the several members present who never attended another meeting, despite his prolific advice on this occasion. The other strange thing about him was his homemade tricycle constructed from two pedal cycle frames, three bicycle wheels and an autocycle engine.

A committee was selected by a geographical process and

among those to serve was a tall thin young man of less than prosperous appearance, wearing a leather flying jacket, whose quiet voice had helped the progress of the meeting all the afternoon. It was obvious that he alone among us had any idea of committee work and meeting organisation and the very first hint of one of the greatest achievements of the ITA came when that quiet voice proposed that a young lady sitting along the row should become our first group treasurer. Garry Nightingale lived in a semi-detached house in Hillingdon and was trying to maintain himself, his home and a small son on a clerical job and an Army pension. The disability pension was for the loss of most of the use of his right arm and leg from wounds received at the Dunkirk evacuation. For employment in a government department in London he travelled daily from Hillingdon in an Argson Runnymede tricycle, of the customary construction with a Villiers 147 cc engine on the back and the refinement of a crude form of pre-selector on the two speed gearbox. This was a system of pins and springs that would change up or down at the operation of the clutch lever. The only concession to the weather was a canvas apron over the knees and the leather flying jacket.

The lady that he nominated as treasurer was Ada and the nomination obviously came as a considerable surprise to her, but that quiet voice pressed on persuasively and Ada went home with two shillings and ninepence to open a Post Office account for us. The 2s 9d was the residue of the 'whip round' held to reimburse Don Booth who had financed the original circulars.

Along with the Committee, the Treasurer and Reg Bolton as secretary, Don was elected as 'group leader', a phrase of the time intended to imply that Mr Booth would lead us all on countless expeditions in the days ahead.

Shortly after the meeting, another circular came round – financed by the 2s 9d in the Post Office – and this was the key to just such a series of expeditions. A long list of places to visit with a meeting place and time, an estimated mileage and return to each place and detailed instructions on how to drive in convoy. Beginning on 5 March with a local tour en route to the first Annual General Meeting of the Association at Edgware, the programme occupied every Saturday afternoon and all day every Sunday throughout the summer months.

The trip to Edgware was a useful exercise in convoy driving and excited little interest in the locality, but once in the schoolroom, we had the first real indoor meeting of members of the Association from all over the country, the first time we had the opportunity to survey many of these noteworthy characters other than when they were sitting in their trikes.

One sign of the times was 'Simmo' – I never found out who he really was – but he was a double amputee and his little leather clad torso rested on a solitary roller skate and his hands paddled him across the floor at break neck speed, accompanied by roller skate noises. When reaching the desired chair, he hoisted his body up on to the chair, parked the skate underneath and the effect of seeing that little legless body whizzing about the hall was forgotten. Another strange sight was the member who turned up wearing a fur coat and a Salvation Army peaked cap, but I never did find out who he was either, but somehow we all soon recognised our Association chairman, Mr Denly who conducted the meeting with an air of confidence that convinced us all that the ITA had really arrived and intended to stay.

The first full scale expedition was in April when all interested parties gathered outside the Wheatsheaf by Bushey Arches in Watford. When Cyril and myself arrived most of the party were assembled, little Bob and the group leader in their Invacars, Harry Kozel in a magnificent Argson Deluxe finished in maroon with lashings of chromium plate on all the fittings and the wheelrims, in which form it served as an advertisement for Argson tricycles and made the rest of us look extremely poor by comparison. Even the Rajah in his howdah was eclipsed by this show piece. Only two ladies turned out that day – Ada and Gwen, who was accompanied by her mother ostensibly to help her start up the engine, but really to take a closer look at the company her daughter was keeping.

It was a dull overcast day in early spring with a general temperature of which we were all very well aware and a threat of rain that made some of us ponder on the wisdom of the day's venture, but the group leader said 'Go', so we all went, just in case something might happen that we would otherwise miss. Up past the Humming Bird to St Albans, where the convoy was drawn up at the traffic lights at the top of Holywell Hill, the steep main street of the town and the cause of a certain amount of bother to us, as some of the two speed machines had to be run back into the kerb to enable their drivers to apply absolutely full throttle for take off on such an incline.

With petrol still on ration, we had the rest of the A5 to ourselves, as we sailed along through Redbourn and Markyate to Dunstable town and the downs beyond and left the main road at Hockliffe to head towards Northampton. Fortune was with us as we passed through Newport Pagnell and made our way eventually into the little town of Olney, where one of a number of stops was made for consultation, this time on the whereabouts of West Street and the bungalow home of Miss Margaret Harris.

Margaret was a wheelchair bound polio and she lived alone in a little bungalow, a degree of independence for a disabled person entirely unknown at that time. There were no structural changes to the building to accept the wheelchair and the front doorway was without steps from the path and the only apparent mechanical aid was a 'helping hand', a sort of long handled gripping device similar to a 'lazy tongs', with which Margaret was able to lift crockery down from the shelves above her reach.

How many hours we spent there that day have faded from memory, but we were there long enough to indulge in a very heated debate about the possibility of there being any honesty in business. It was a case of Dave Marsland, the Rajah, against the rest and there were no winners, but the town of Olney certainly knew that something unusual had happened there that day.

It was a very long journey home, as strange roads always make journeys long and even longer when those roads are deserted, but when I reached Wembley, I was very thankful and gave little thought to that other dozen miles to Wimbledon that Cyril had to take that night.

Driving in the dark was somewhat perilous as an open tricycle such as we had would be capable of as much as 40 mph providing you did not hit a bump at that speed, whence you could easily be thrown out of the machine and the lighting for locating such bumps in the dark was very grim. A small headlamp mounted above the front forks was fed directly from the generator in the flywheel of the engine and the degree of illumination varied with the revs of the engine and it was not until you reached maximum revs that any appreciable illumination appeared at all, and at tick over the light was barely visible.

Come Whit Monday 1949, we met at the War Memorial, Isleworth, and set off towards Kingston and the A24, but I did not recognise Leatherhead as the signposts such as had been erected after the war – they were all removed with the intention of confusing an invader – led us on to the Leatherhead By-Pass round the town and on to Dorking, Horsham and eventually the back road up on to Devil's Dyke. This was a desolate windswept area of tarmac with one or two pillboxes facing the sea and in this chilly atmosphere, we met the Sussex group of the ITA and we posed for a newspaper photographer fully wrapped up in leather flying jackets and every other item of protection we could muster.

One or two drivers failed to make the steep climb up to the Dyke and they were the only ones among us who saw the sea that day as they drove on down to the front, before we all set out home again after one of the very first inter–group meetings of the ITA. It was always interesting to meet folk from other parts in this way and many friendships evolved from these meetings, but Devil's Dyke was a long and tiring journey and chugging homewards it began to get dark. It was on just such occasions as this that the adoration that Gwen always showed for Don Booth would begin to wilt, not because of the darkness, but for the fear she felt for the paternal reception that awaited her when she arrived home in Bushey after the curfew hour.

Apprehension was high in most households as they sat waiting to hear that trike roar up the road after one of our planned marathon trips, but in Gwen's household, her father would be out pacing the street waiting to deliver dire threats of a depth related directly to the lateness of the hour. Her fear of these encounters was considerable and for this reason alone, she developed a strange belief that I was the only one who could be depended upon to really know the way home from anywhere, a belief that was quite unfounded. So it was that as darkness or the traffic lights or other obstacles divided our party, that Gwen would abandon poor old Don and stick limpetlike to the tatty little rearlight of my 'Argson' and eventually we would reach home, but certainly no sooner than Don, although possibly by a different route.

It was on one of these evenings like the return from Devil's Dyke that we entered Kingston-upon-Thames in darkness and I made for the only road I then knew that led out of Kingston towards Richmond – Lower Ham Road – that passed between the gas works and a power station and at that time was open to through traffic. Several trikes followed me between those daunting industrial edifices along by Canonbury Gardens and suddenly out on to the river bank. A vast expanse of dark and chilly water, a narrow road with occasional gas lamps and our own puny illuminations on the front of each trike doing very little to help keep us to the road. We reached home safely but there were subsequent murmurings about the incident.

The runs went on throughout the summer of 1949 and we all travelled to so many places that alone few of us would have considered visiting. Box Hill, where you could park on the grass by the viewing point and sit there all day without another soul arriving to spoil the tranquility. Epping Forest was much the same, although the odd bus route straddled the area and brought a few people out on Sundays. Hindhead was visited once and Burnham Beeches and the river at Runnymede were frequent destinations. Some very rigid rules were issued to members attending these runs, rules which could not possibly work in practice, such as the bold statement that the 'leader will pull up every hour to enable the stragglers to catch up'. Mechanical failure was such that it was impossible to keep the whole party going for a whole hour and the chief cause was the carbon bridge forming across the points of the huge 18 mm spark plugs with which most of the trikes were fitted and long spells were spent removing cooked plugs and fitting one you would select from your spare collection of half a dozen or more in your tool bag. At every scheduled stop there would be sessions of dismantling these dirty plugs – they were a form of screw-together assembly – and cleaning them meticulously with a wire brush and fine emery paper before placing them in the collection ready for the next emergency halt on the road.

Another very good reason why the aforementioned rule

was impractical was the time honoured call of nature which always seemed to call more frequently on the ladies than it did on the men.

'Alright for you men', they would say, 'you can go behind a hedge!'

Many carried a glass receptacle and some were none too concerned about where they would pull up to use it, but alas with the ladies with awkward disabilities, it was a constant hunt for toilets and they had to be convenient conveniences as well before they had any hope of gaining comfort.

We paid a return visit to Margaret Harris in Olney later in the summer and the company that day included Emily Russ, a dear little lady in her early sixties and Emily was driving a very small Harding tricycle with a single speed 98 cc engine under the seat. Flat out it was capable of very little more than 15 mph which meant that Emily was holding up the convoy. But she pressed on valiantly and so valiantly did she press on that after driving along King Harry Lane to avoid Holywell Hill in St Albans, we continued down by the village pond at the back of the town to emerge on to the A5 main road and there it was that poor Emily took the corner at an excessive speed and ended up in the gutter on the far side of the A5 with the trike upside down on top of her.

The speed with which a policeman, an AA patrol and an ambulance arrived was truly remarkable. The constable took details down in his little book, the AA man moved the trike into a nearby garage and the ambulance took Emily to hospital where she was found to be little worse for her experience. Given a rest and a cup of tea, she was then taken back to her trike and she drove home alone to Edgware.

The rest of the party went on to Whipsnade and later in the evening they were making their way home when the need for petrol – we had the coupons, if not the cash – became apparent and thus we all arrived on the forecourt of the very same garage where Emily's trike had been stored. Some of us took petrol and others sat there chatting to a young constable, a man new to the force who was then following up the details and outcome of that morning's drama. He explained the rules of police procedure and he seemed a little bored with the tedium of his task, but this soon passed by as Gwen came tottering across the forecourt and enquired if there was a ladies' comfort station there. The constable was equal to the situation as he conveyed the unhappy message to Gwen that the ladies' toilet was at the far end of the garage, a very long and laborious walk for her, but right here was the gents' and the constable immediately disappeared inside to ascertain that no males were lurking therein, before emerging to announce, 'This way, madam, I will guard the door.' We all sat round and waited and as the highly embarrassed and greatly relieved Gwen emerged from the gents' there was a great roar of welcome on the garage forecourt and that story was related in many a home that night.

During the summer months of 1949, the ITA organised its very first overseas rally to Zutphen in Holland. The large party that set out by trike for Harwich included Gwen and Ada, the trikes were conveyed by the railway steamer without charge and were landed at Hook of Holland where the full extent of the welcome was first shown. So soon after the war there was still bitterness felt for Germany and a corresponding fondness for Britain, which gave our party a police motorcycle escort to all the interesting places in Holland, including the Arnhem cemetery and to numerous civic receptions in many different Dutch towns. Perhaps I have regretted that I did not go along on this fabulous trip, but when our two members arrived home afterwards they were in an unenviable state of joyous exhaustion. A truly wonderful time had been had by all!

Plans were in hand for the second national rally in Richmond Park when Don received a letter from the national secretary conveying details of the proposed programme for the rally. A new idea had been dreamed up by the organisers and they were asking us in Middlesex Group to put the idea into practice and this snippet of information was read to a meeting of the group by Don in his official capacity. It was suggested that we should perform a display of formation driving as part of the afternoon's entertainment, a sort of very unmusical musical ride and would someone please work out the formation patterns, collect together a team and train them all in the timing and maneouvres.

I have no idea what thoughts were in my mind when I raised my hand as that volunteer. I had no experience of organising anything and no real idea of what was wanted, but this was a classic example of the real value of the ITA. It put you on the spot and more or less forced you, or shamed you, into achievements that you would never have considered yourself capable of without that encouragement.

I went home from that meeting in a very worried state. I had said I would do it and so I would have to do it, but I still had little idea of how to do it, but with the passage of the days, the ideas and the possibilities came to mind, generated by necessity and encouraged by the volunteers anxious to help.

We secured the use of Fryent School playground on which to practise and the team of eight with no reserves was mustered with six Argsons, one Invacar and one Tippen, a breed then just beginning to appear as Ministry of Health issue under the National Health Act of the previous year. The team included the ladies, Gwen, Ada and Marion Luker, the only person to have a crude form of self starter on her tricycle and a gadget that clanged away like a town hall clock every time the button was pressed.

The round and round, the scissors movements, the line abreast and the peeling off to start again, all went along quite well and everyone turned up one evening a week to practise. On the Saturday before the rally Sunday we were able to have a full rehearsal on the parade ground in Richmond Park. It was a great relief to me to know that we could actually do the full routine without mishap or mistake, but the only onlookers were the servicemen left on camp for the weekend and not the full crowd we expected to turn up on Sunday. We did many complete runs through that afternoon and we only gave up on the suggestion that there might be tea about and tea there certainly was, served to us by the cookhouse orderly in a galvanised bucket, followed by a hand out of cups!

We drove home that evening reasonably happy about our rehearsal and without too much worry about tomorrow which dawned bright and sunny and drew us all back to Richmond Park by ten o'clock in the morning. This was a great day for renewing acquaintances of the year before and cementing friendships then established. There were the people from the Sussex group whom we met on Devil's Dyke at Whitsun and the so called 'twins' from the Surrey group,

Gladys and Eleanor, two unrelated young women who both lived in Epsom and who generated most of the steam and a certain amount of hysteria that kept the Surrey group going. Gladys had a lesser disability, wearing one massive brown boot to equalise ambulations, but Eleanor's problems were more complicated as the aftermath of a brittle bone structure, but both drove Argson 'Runnymede' tricycles and their exuberance was such that they did not really need a group of the ITA to encourage them to greater mobility.

From the North West of England came that little band of tricyclists who booked in for a couple of nights at The Peahen in St Albans and such like places which led some of us to believe, quite mistakenly, that they were very wealthy, but the probable answer was that they sank all in the need for accessible accommodation within striking distance of Richmond Park. Leader of this party was a very softly spoken, ponderous young man in a wheelchair, who lived in the very un-Peahen town of Rochdale. His name was Fred Needham and it was Fred that in years to come was to replace Denny as the National Chairman of the DDA.

The programme for the day was a series of heats in the egg and spoon races, obstacle races and other competitions of this kind, a grand and very noisy parade of everyone after lunch with Denny taking the salute as we all drove in endless procession, several trikes abreast. This was followed by the finals, a demonstration by the myriad manufacturers of that day and at last our ceremonial manoeuvres by the Middlesex team were on. We drove in single file down the centre of the cleared arena and peeled off alternately left and right to drive round the edges close to the crowds of people sitting on the park chairs that marked the boundary and this led on to all the other movements that made this display, never before performed by invalid tricycles, into the spectacular that brought a fair old round of applause from our audience. It was a great relief when it was successfully completed and it was then that I knew that my five shilling subscription had really done something for me.

The rest of the summer programme saw us tearing off in all directions every weekend in any weather and the effects of sitting in a bucket seat with an apron over your knees and a weatherproof coat on, was usually to fill the bottom of the bucket up with water every time it rained in a respectable manner and this process was distinctly uncomfortable particularly if there was a long drive home ahead of you – and there usually was.

On one of these days Garry approached me wearing that sad look of intense concentration that told me he was planning another master stroke of organisation. In his hand was a foolscap book about half an inch thick with a motif on the front cover that told of its origins. He handed the book to me, it contained lined pages awaiting entry and he said in his quiet purposeful manner,

'You can take the minutes!'

I remained blissfully unaware of what he meant and answered quite innocently,

'What are minutes?'

The first factual, starchy lesson began immediately and soon I was installed at committee meetings to record the discussion and decisions of that committee, a task, that by chance, was to lead to greater things.

Finance was becoming a pressing problem within the group as the membership had to be circulated with a newsletter on some regular basis and the Secretary was required to answer his own correspondence and fan mail and make the necessary arrangements for some of our journeys and so it was that Garry produced the unoriginal idea of running a sweepstake on the St Leger. This proposal was immediately jumped upon by the association's officers who were still endeavouring to maintain the ITA as a subscription organisation without subsidiary fund raising powers, but it was evident that we could not run the group successfully on these lines and Garry was very keen on his idea of a St Leger Draw, so we set up a subsidiary organisation to raise our subsidiary funds for us, with the imposing title of the Middlesex Invalid Tricycle Social Club.

When the tickets were printed and delivered, it came as a bit of a shock to me to find that as Minutes Secretary I had become Secretary of the MITS Club, and subsequently the proclaimed organiser of the St Leger Draw and my name and address appeared on every ticket.

I don't quite know who actually did do the organisation, I only know it was not me, but the thoroughness of the details left little doubt in my mind and when the race was run and the winners paid out, the group had put £219 into the bank as a stock pile for future needs. This sum was considerably more than the National Association could muster and so it was that eventually the ITA itself became a registered charity which meant that the group could run fund raising events in the Association name, the MITS Club was wound up and I was left alone to write in my Minutes Book.

The next great idea for raising funds came from Gwen, when she announced that her sister was prepared to organise a Jumble Sale in Bushey in aid of the spare tricycle fund. This fund was a cherished ideal in the Taylor household when Gwen was in constant mechanical trouble and like so many of us, her employment depended on the trike being on the road. So with her Girl Guide sister, Enid, making use of the Boy Scout motto 'Be Prepared', we all set to, to collect the wherewithal to hold our jumble sale in Bushey Congregational Church Hall in the autumn of 1949.

Most of the accumulated junk was stored in the Taylor household and somehow everything was shipped to the hall for the Saturday afternoon sale and before a door was opened, a considerable queue of customers, honest and otherwise, had formed outside, which surprised and encouraged us. It was a tremendous afternoon's fun and a great education to see the items that some people were over anxious to acquire and the stories of individual transactions went on for weeks, but one of the best concerned the zealous gentleman who came to help that afternoon and when he met a lady from the village in the hall, he jested that she might be interested in buying a particularly fine perambulator that we had for sale. The lady bristled immediately and rebuked our helper with a venomous tongue before stepping aside to reveal that her companion was her daughter, who was in imminent need of a perambulator. Our zealous and embarrassed helper retired from the shop floor to partake of a cup of tea to help restore his enthusiasm.

The battle raged all afternoon and a strange ferretty little man who arrived as a customer and endeavoured to establish himself as a salesman during the foray, eventually emerged as the man who made an over modest offer for the tremendous residue of junk that lay scattered across the hall. What he did with several sacks full of old shoes, we do not know, but the clothing and some other items were readily disposable in the junk yard in Watford in exchange for a small sum of money, a facility of which we were unable to avail ourselves as we had no adequate transport of our own.

While the helpers sat back to yarn over their tea and generally recover from the extraordinary experience of running a jumble sale in a Hertfordshire village, the departing customers were enjoying their own hilarious experiences of carting their spoils homewards.

On Clay Hill in Bushey stands the village police station from which numerous policemen proceed on their various beats around the parish or manor and just as one such earnest constable set out in his newly polished boots to wend his way down Clay Hill, there came the lusty roar of an Argson tricycle being pressed to its limits to ensure that it would make the steep gradient of the hill without faltering. But falter it did, for carried upon that tricycle, in addition to the driver, was a Victorian tailor's dummy. The round wooden base tucked under his feet, the long polished centre pole lay beside him and the busty torso section to which my grandmother had fitted numerous of her Victorian style dresses during manufacture in years gone by, nestled comfortably on the driver's knees with its 'cut off at the hips' end resting on his feet. As the constable and the trike approached each other, a sudden bump in the road dislodged that busty torso and it rolled off into the gutter.

The British policeman is a legend of helpful discretion and so our constable hastened to assist in the distress of our friend.

'You've dropped something, Sir,' he said and back came the instant reply,

'It's all right officer, it's only the body!'

Thirty-five pounds went into the bank after that afternoon's escapade and the thoughts of a spare trike seemed a little brighter for those of us with mechanical worries.

Through the dark cold days of winter it was not possible or practical to run outdoor meetings and there were some worries about holding the group together until the better weather would allow a resumption of our travels, but Don managed to keep everyone circulated with a duplicated news sheet which keyed everyone up with the great plans for next year and the quarterly copies of the national magazine, the *Magic Carpet* continued to arrive on time. There were a few odd private meetings between some of the membership and the committee was meeting every month, usually in the home of Dave Marsland in Harrow, to hammer out the organisation of our future programme. High on the list of those plans came an Annual Dinner, a project to which Garry was particularly devoted and to which he insisted there should be no charge to our members. This was a very controversial point, but after much heated discussion and a great deal of work by the appointed organiser, Ada Nichols, the grand evening arrived and everyone connected with the group, together with a few who were not, were there in Kerswell's restaurant at Eastcote.

Speeches were made by Don, who seemed to be in his element and by Denny in his official capacity as National Chairman of the ITA on an occasion that must have proved to him that his Association had really arrived and established itself. The evening's entertainment which followed was of a very high order indeed and so it should have been, as the four solo artists to perform had cost us the princely sum of £20 between them. The total cost of our first annual dinner made a deep rut in our bank balance and the self congratulation about the success of the dinner was tempered with doubts about our economic standing. But our first Annual General Meeting passed by with general approval of a summer programme that was to be almost a repeat of 1949 with one or two notable exceptions.

During the early days of the war I had met Roy on the hospital ward in Stanmore and a spasmodic friendship grew between us. Early in 1950 Roy called in at Barnhill Road with his MOH Tippen to be told by my mother that I was out with the group and she promptly enrolled him as a member of the ITA. When Roy expressed an interest in coming to our first Annual Dinner at Eastcote, my mother suggested that we invite Roy and one or two other members home to a brief introduction for him. Thus it was that Cyril, Gwen and Marion met Roy for the first time in Barnhill Road. Roy lost no time in escorting Gwen and Marion back to Bushey that night when Gwen's father was over enthusiastic with his welcome. 'Come as often as you like, boy', he said, and Roy was there every night till a late hour for long afterwards. In

1952 they were married at Bushey Congregational Church, the scene of our jumble sales and the marriage lasted for fourteen years but sadly ended in divorce.

The idea of a weekend away was greeted with enthusiasm and work was immediately put in hand to plan accommodation for a party over the Whitsun weekend. A lot of debate ensued on possible venues, but snags kept arising and our sights were re-focussed to bring Billy Butlin into view, as chalet accommodation would at least be at ground level and toilet blocks would hopefully be accessible.

The Butlin camp chosen for our weekend away was at Clacton and negotiations were entered into that culminated in a highly successful weekend for us, if not quite so successful for Mr Butlin. On the Friday afternoon before the Whitsun weekend, many of us sneaked away from our work to meet up in small parties and wend our way out across Essex towards the chilly briny of the east coast. It was on this journey with my weekend bag aboard the Argson that I turned into a garage to purchase petrol – at 2s 1½d per gallon – and when I held out my coupons, the pump attendant made a very uncalled for remark that was very rude indeed, but it took me some little time to realise that petrol rationing had ceased that very afternoon and that my treasured coupon collection was worthless.

Clacton seemed a terrible long way on strange roads but at last we drove into the Butlin Camp and were ushered into the fish and chip bar where portions were served with ketchup before we fell back in our trikes to drive round the camp looking for chalet numbers. This was but the first circuit of the camp by those noisy trikes and it seemed that throughout the evening and most of the night, there would be someone somewhere driving a trike round the camp, which did not endear us to our fellow campers or to Mr Butlin's Redcoats.

Everyone spent the evenings as they wished, watching the dancing in the ballroom, drinking in the bar or viewing the town's amenities, but everyone gathered together for the Show on Saturday evening. During the afternoon everyone with their trikes was lined up in front of the Butlin ballroom for an official photograph to be taken and it is only from this photograph that we really know just how many people did go to join in our first weekend away. Among the party was Bill

Powell, a middle–aged undistinguished man who never wasted valuable drinking time, but who drove an elderly tiller steered Argson trike at not inconsiderable speeds and it was Bill on whom the photographer's eye alighted for his next Butlin publicity photograph that could have been the highlight of poor old Bill's life. A scantily clad Butlin Beauty was whistled up to sit on the side of the trike seat while Bill's left arm settled in place around her loins and her photographer shouted, 'Hold it!' He did!

The next episode was tricycle hockey on the big beautiful grassland in the centre of the chalets. There were no rules, everyone except myself joined in and a tremendous noise rose with the great cloud of two stroke smoke making play almost impossible, but everyone continued to tear round and round until the final whistle and not until then was the state of the pitch considered at all, by which time it was too late. The grass had been cut to pieces and everyone retired from the scene with discreet haste.

I shared a chalet with an ambulatory 'spondi' who somehow managed to sleep in the top bunk, unless he slept in the chair – I never really found out which and neither did I find out what happened when he went for a prowl around well after dark. His physical condition belied the avowed intent of his expedition so no–one was likely to have come to very much harm by his marauding, but while he was away, I rolled into the bottom bunk and then made the mistake of sitting up in bed. The bunks were wooden framed wartime structures with wiremesh under the mattress and when I sat up, my head more than touched the underside of the top bunk and my hair became entangled in the mesh above me, leaving me in a half sitting up position which my spinal deformity did not take kindly to, and which required the full use of both my arms to prevent myself falling backwards and tearing my hair out by the roots. The return of my chalet companion was very welcome.

We all drove home on Sunday afternoon and it was then that we saw the first signs of the end of our freedom on the road as everyone else could now buy the petrol that would afford them the miles of motoring that we had all enjoyed in such solitude on the roads of Britain in 1949.

8

To Imitate Success

Nothing would ever be the same again and our efforts to repeat the previous season's programme in 1950 was an example of the folly of trying to imitate success, but the trips hither and thither went on and the irrepressible Don came up with some new ideas following the derationing of petrol.

Silverstone was just beginning its transition from a wartime airfield to a racing circuit and Don was a great motor racing fan. So it was that ten of us set out again on the A5 and followed Don up to the traffic jam that spread for miles around the lanes in the Silverstone area. We joined the jam of cars for a few minutes and nothing seemed to move anywhere and the sky did not look too happy either, so Don pulled out to the offside of the road and we all fell in behind and the little trail of trikes set off at caution along the wrong side of the lanes, thus we drove for many miles passing an endless queue of stationary motor cars all intent on getting in to see the British Grand Prix on this new racing track.

There was nothing but the grass and the concrete perimeter track there at the time, no grandstands, fencing, entrance gates or crowd control and no one seemed to take much notice of us and certainly Don didn't seem to take much notice of anyone else as we drove straight on to the course to take up a vantage point that was strictly too near to the track, but which afforded us a spectacular view of the ERAs, Alfa Romeos and Maseratis as they battled for places in the British Grand Prix.

There were two other visits to Silverstone in the same year to see motor cycle racing in both the 'Hutchinson 100' and 'Motor Cycling Saturday' but access to the course on both

72

occasions was much easier as the majority of spectators were motor cycle mounted and there were virtually no jams at all. For one of these events we were all parked by Stowe Corner from where we could see the approaching pack of motor bikes, the tactics on the bend and away down the straight. The sidecar racing was very spectacular with British and foreign machines competing, but this was the day of the rise of Geoff Duke as a motor cycle ace and we were to see a previous reigning champion come a sensational cropper.

The pack, including Duke and Harold Daniel, came hammering into Stowe Corner, the loudspeaker commentary estimating the cornering speed as 70 mph, when one bike went over and machine and rider went into strange gyrations down the track with the bike a clear leader over the flailing body. It was Harold Daniel and we were completely astonished to see him get to his feet and be helped away by marshalls who were soon on the scene. There must be a lesson in road safety here somewhere.

These were three grand days out in that year, days that Don and myself particularly enjoyed and it was one of those days that nearly brought its own disaster to us as well, for on the way home from Silverstone, a halt was called to check that everyone was still roadworthy. I was sitting there minding my own business just waiting for the convoy to close up, when there came a terrific kick in the pants that sent me up the road at some speed, as hand brakes were frail and conserved for vital use only. The cause of the impact was our worthy Secretary who, for reasons best known to himself, chose to use me as the sand-drag or buffer stops for retardation. He seemed quite happy about it until someone said, 'Are your front forks meant to be back there?'

The single legs of the forks had bent back just below the bottom links of the spring mounting and this gave the driver a very difficult drive home to Harrow.

On another sporting occasion, we met on a wet Sunday morning at Canons Park roundabout and set out for St Albans and the A6 northwards through Harpenden, with our minds set on Luton Hoo, the Werner home in Bedfordshire where a speed trial was scheduled for that day. We turned off the A6 and were soon in the grounds of Luton Hoo, where Don led onwards along the roads through those extensive grounds, when a marshall indicated that we should turn into a parking area, but Don declined with thanks as this was a quagmire of mud and promptly drove on. We all trailed along behind on the right hand side of the road as the left was lined with the most beautiful selection of vintage sports cars that one could wish to see – ERAs, Bugattis, Amilcars, Bentleys, Vauxhalls and the rest were all viewed with great interest until a marshall hurriedly ordered us up on to the grass bank and off the roadway. We lined up beside the road and faced the cars just where a large banner was flying proclaiming the start. The cars we had inspected were all lined up for the individual stop watch start and we were there with a ringside seat, albeit in the rain, as each competitor clipped the time clock gadget with his front wheel and the marshall was required to remove it before the rear wheel ran over it also, which called for great dexterity.

The course was up the lane through the grounds to a turning circle where an oil drum marked the centre and each car in turn had to be hurled round this oil drum and hurtle back to the start and finish line. Only as the first competitor came home did we realise that we had, moments before, been driving serenely along the 'run-off' road for the event, calmly unaware of what might have been coming towards us at breakneck speed.

It was an enjoyable afternoon as the weather improved and the line of vintage machinery moved slowly forward to its turn to show its paces, when the largest competitor of all, a massive touring Mercedes of the 1930s, with a two stage supercharger drew up to the line. The sun-bespectacled driver sat motionless gazing skyward for a long time and Cyril turned to me and yelled above the noise of the revving engines, 'He's praying to Allah!' and well he might have been, but how he got round that oil drum, we never knew.

All the escapades of those days were dutifully catalogued and described in the subsequent pages of the Middlesex group newsletter *Mrs Frequently* which viewed from a distance make unbelievable reading today. Dave Marsland was now honorary Treasurer and the annual audit of the books was carried out by Cyril Porter and Bob Laughlin as we were not then obliged to have accredited auditors. The particular operation took a very long time and after repeatedly wading through the accounts which failed to balance and always by the same sum of money, the baffled auditors faced the portly figure of the treasurer, who then produced another receipt for exactly the sum that was unaccounted for. There is no record of the ensuing conversation, but we can safely assume the acid content.

During all this time the Argson continued to carry me on most of our expeditions and also on my daily couple of miles to work in the Exhibition Grounds, but on the odd occasion I was very pleased to be able to borrow one of the strange machines bequeathed to the group as 'spare tricycles'. We never did actually buy a spare tricycle, but rather did we depend on one of our members to expire, whence his family would offer his machine to us for just such a use. All very morbid, but quite a practical solution from both sides of the transaction since the market for invalid tricycles had dwindled away following the grand issue by the Ministry of Health to most of the potential customers.

That same Ministry of course, were now also paying for the manufacture and repair of that ghastly set of structural steelwork that I was obliged to assemble around myself each morning. The design of this contraption had advanced not one visible millimetre since pre-war years and was still very weighty, decidedly uncomfortable and an unbearable restriction on my every movement. An immense strain was placed on this equipment whenever I locked myself out straight and raised myself to the standing position and again when I had to lie heavily on the starting handle of the Argson. Rivets slackened back, steelwork fractured and leather straps or covering split, which usually meant digging out an obsolete set of callipers, dusting them down and applying them to the person at even greater discomfort to myself, so that I could set out in the Argson for Stanmore in the hope of having a repair made in the least possible time, although often over a span of some weeks.

The more interesting range of manufacture of course, was the invalid tricycle and at each successive ITA rally, the respective manufacturers were invited to demonstrate their products before us all. Many weird and wonderful machines were shown to us in this section prior to the Ministry of Health taking an active part in tricycle design, but at the 1950 rally in Richmond Park, the first Ministry inspired creation was paraded before us by the AC Car Company from Thames Ditton. A real three-wheeled car with a tiny dumpling front wheel, two big wire rear wheels hidden under valances, an all over body faired down at the front into a single head lamp, built up at the back to provide a full height boot for a wheelchair, a double-fold door on the nearside only and a black canvas hood that could be screwed down to the chromium windscreen frame. Celluloid sidescreens completed the structure which was all finished in a tasteful shade of polychromatic honeysuckle with chromium bumpers fore and aft.

We all ogled at this new vision of the future and the demonstration was brought to a climax by laying a dozen timbers out like railway sleepers in miniature and driving the new vehicle straight over the lot without a murmur – we had indeed got suspension that would deal with the bumps, but this raised the hackles of a rival manufacturer who immediately drove his own unsprung machine straight at the timbers. Momentum carried him over the first two or three, but he was then forced to retire as he could make no further progress on this trail which only served to draw attention to the difference in the products. After the demonstration everyone was busy telling everyone else, 'Of course, you'll never get one of those!' but time alone would tell.

The group activities continued as before with much the same enthusiasm. Another St Leger draw was run and another Jumble Sale organised at Bushey by Gwen and Enid and slight animosity between Garry and Dave Marsland continued until Dave resigned as Treasurer and the resourceful Garry cast his eye far and wide among the membership for a possible replacement. From the rule book of the Association, he read again the line about not more than two Associate members to serve on any one committee, which set him thinking about Associate members as possible Treasurers and the Jumble Sale brought Enid Taylor to his mind. So it was that the quiet persuasive Garry charm talked Enid into accepting the treasurership with no voting rights as an Associate member.

Our second Annual Dinner was arranged at the Century Hotel in Wembley Park in February 1951 and the notable thing about the date was the arrival of my very first 'Ministry' trike. The bespectacled little man with the sandy hair and the cheery grin drove up in the brown AC, all beautifully polished and clean. He removed his trade plates, gave me superficial instruction on the controls of the vehicle, patted the bodywork almost with affection and said

'She's all yours!' before setting out on the long walk back to public transport at Wembley Park station to begin his journey home to Thames Ditton.

I viewed this new monster with some disbelief; there it stood with its beautiful shining polychromatic honeysuckle paintwork, its hood down and its luxurious shoulder high seat behind the aircraft steering wheel, just waiting for me to climb aboard – and it had cost me not one bean! It was sometime before I eventually opened the door and lowered myself into the single seat of this machine that was to change so many things in my life ahead. I opened the double fold door again, heaved my feet over the side of the seat extension flap that would invite passenger carrying and removed the backrest of the seat with the panel behind and peered into the works.

The Beesa 250 stood at the back, almost under the seat a large Burman gearbox with the multiplate clutch on the side and between these two units was another cast alloy box from which the half shafts spread sideways to the back wheels. This was the differential and all were connected by transmission chains; from the engine forward to the gear box a very long chain indeed and back from there to the differential, a short chain; it all looked very impressive after the Argson.

The suspension, so effectively demonstrated in Richmond Park, was clearly soft and pliable as the vehicle sank down when you applied your body weight to it and peering deeper into the works it was possible to detect the big square tubular backbone of the frame from which everything stemmed, including three cross tubes just under the seat, from the ends of which were hung the trailing arms carrying the rear wheels that bounced up and down under long coil springs. Across the top of the differential box was fitted another cross tube that swept upwards at each end to form an anchor point for the two springs and their appropriate dampers and perched on top of the centre of that cross tube, a belt driven dynamo, and there was a corresponding ammeter to tell you what it was doing.

I replaced the metal panel and the strange tubular gadget held there by Terry clips, put the seat cushion back in place and drew my feet aboard again to study the driving technique. The aircraft wheel had a centre horn button and the two horns of the wheel stood vertically, the left hand one was fitted with a twist grip for the throttle and on the right hand one, a plain rubber grip. Ahead of the twist grip, a massive cast lever that could be drawn up to the grip by stretching out the three fingers of my left hand, so disengaging the clutch and the wheel itself could be rotated through 180° lock to lock, controlled by a steering box immediately behind the dashboard. To the right of the seat on the non-exit side of the trike was a large gated gear change lever that moved fore and aft and attached to this lever, another cable operating lever also to work the clutch via a link mechanism under the seat. Also under the seat was the battery and another cross tube that stuck out each side of the seat box where each end turned forward in a horizontal plane to form a lever that could be pulled upward to apply the cable operated brakes. The left hand lever was unusable but the right hand lever was fitted up with a press-in button on the end that would engage in a ratchet when needed for parking. Otherwise you would place your thumb on the gear shift gate, wrap your fingers round the brake lever and heave upwards to provide very sensitive and positive braking while the left hand remained on the wheel and pulled the clutch lever too.

A car type electric starter motor was supplemented with a long hand lever also beside the seat and linked to the kick start spindle of the gearbox and the petrol supply was gravity fed with a tap.

I put up the hood, slotted in the sidescreens and laid back in that deep luxurious seat, to drool over the snug, dry, comfort of it all compared to the rigours of the Argson, that I might now be able to retire from regular use.

For eight eventful years and 50,000 marvellous miles, the brown AC was mine and in that time the tales of mechanical mishap would be a story on its own, but experience taught me how to deal with most of the problems such as carrying a bicycle pump to remove water from the distributor and that other bedevilment, the air-locking of the petrol supply, when the rolling motion of the trike on corners would uncover the petrol outlet from the tank and allow air into the pipe. The cure to this was diplomacy, as you had to accost a likely passerby and tactfully ask him if he would mind removing the petrol cap situated on the top of the body, apply his lips to the inlet and blow like mad, a most distasteful exercise for anyone, but it was surprising how many people there were doing this all over the country at the time.

Typical of these instances was my involuntary pause outside the Lancaster Hotel when, as a bus passed slowly by, the conductor stepped off the back, banged on the bus which stopped, and then came back to offer assistance – by blowing into the petrol tank! On another occasion we came to rest whilst circumnavigating Hyde Park Corner as it was then and almost immediately an *Evening News* van drew up beside me in the middle of the road, the driver stepped out and pushed me on to the centre island before leaping back into his van and tearing off on his round.

The most difficult situation I encountered was the day I stopped involuntarily outside a small estate known as Pilgrims Way, when one of the residents leapt over the fence with a bottle in his hand yelling 'This'll make it go!' I had great difficulty in restraining him from pouring a pint of white spirit into my petrol tank.

The stories are numerous and so were some of the built-in problems of the trike, as the carburettor was mounted directly in line above the silencer, the petrol feed pipe was not clipped up to the body but laid on the engine cowling and there was no adequate tensioning medium for that long chain, a failing which eventually showed up in the Bayswater Road when the back nearside settled down on to the wheel and did not rise again. Inspection showed that the chain had chewed away at the cross tube carrying the rear springs and the tube had fractured lowering the body on to the tyre.

A similar thing happened on the front end after years of service. A motor cycle style headstock was held to the square tube backbone frame by two large bolts passing horizontally through the headstock casting and engaging in four lugs on the square tube and when the lower lugs parted from the frame, the forks, trailing arms and wheel moved forward of the machine, lowering the nose of the trike on to the road from where it did not rise.

Another built-in problem came from the engine adaptations where a main shaft extension carried a dynamo pulley and a big aluminium flywheel to which the starter ring was fixed and on the face were cast the cooling fan blades. This flywheel was mounted on a steel boss and fixed there by large rivets, but what a shame the rivets were soft and the flywheel became slightly loose after a good hammering by the starter motor kick, thus upsetting the balance of the engine.

Such were the problems that fortunes were made by repair contractors rectifying these faults and a few extra faults for luck.

Not that the trike problems were paramount, for the miles of happy travel were many and every mile was a joy in the well sprung comfort of the AC with the hood up or down as the weather dictated. In the plans for 1951 it was agreed to try another Whitsun weekend and this was eventually established at St Mary's Bay near Dymchurch in a bungalow hotel on this rather uninspiring coastline.

Skipping work again on Friday afternoon, we set out in some sort of convoy across London and out towards Maidstone on the A20 through the Kent countryside around Tenterden and Biddenden and at long last into St Mary's Bay. When we arose on Saturday morning plans were made to visit Winchelsea, Rye and Hastings and the collection of trikes showed an increasing number of ACs in the ranks, the smaller machines being abandoned one by one as more and more people climbed 'two-up' into the ACs, a practice which led the Ministry to fit small notices on the dashboards saying 'No passenger carrying allowed', but it was too late for this weekend. As the line of ACs and a few open trikes prepared to move off, one lonely figure remained, that of our one Associate member who came by train for the weekend, Enid Taylor. It was Doris Beard who spoke up with a solution, as she noted the only AC without a passenger was mine and that was soon rectified before we began a most enjoyable trip round the Winchelsea, Rye and Hastings area of Sussex.

The whole weekend was very pleasant and successful and included a trip by the whole party on the Romney, Hythe and Dymchurch Railway, for which purpose the train was lengthened by the addition of more rolling stock. Why we all elected to travel out to the wilderness of Dungeness on a Sunday afternoon is problematical but the two return tickets I bought for that trip are still with me today, as a reminder of my appreciation of the company I was happy to keep and as a means of dating the photograph we had taken with the AC on the main road in Sandgate that weekend.

During the summer months we spent our Wednesday evenings on the public enclosure of Northolt Airport, then in use for all European flights by British European Airways and some foreign airlines.

This put quite a strain on the AC after its little 'cakewalk' round to the factory in Exhibition Grounds each day, as after tea we headed off to Bushey to do a little more illicit passenger carrying by collecting Enid on the seat extension flap so thoughtfully provided by the Ministry of Health. The vehicle was forty inches wide overall and the big Dunlopillo seat was in the centre with this wooden extension flap to fill the other ten or twelve inches between the seat and the door of the trike, which had to be firmly closed after any passenger came aboard.

Thus loaded we set off towards Northwood and Ruislip to reach the airport enclosure and spend an enjoyable and informative evening in the company of the group. The Dakotas and the Vikings flew in with monotonous regularity from all over Europe and now and then might come some less familiar flying machine to add a little variety before dusk came and we all set off for home, in my case via Bushey.

The summer passed pleasantly and there were countless trips out and always in the old AC but not always in the company of the group. Such was the day that I took Enid to Baughurst on one of my fairly regular trips to visit my Aunt and Uncle, but not without some mishap, that loomed up on the Denham Bypass when a loud tinkling noise was accompanied by a total lack of charge on the ammeter.

We pulled in, removed the high backrest cushion and the inspection panel behind and peered into the works. The belt hung limply from the dynamo pulley with its far end attached to nothing as the driving pulley had disappeared. With great good fortune the AA man appeared just at the critical moment and he retrieved the pulley, the compression spring, the locking washer and the nut from the respective positions along the road behind us. With the AA man in the boot and myself leaning through the inspection panel, we just managed to compress the spring so that the nut could be started and this time the locking washer was properly locked in place and we were ready for the off. As passenger carrying was now forbidden and we were doubtful where the AA man stood in this dilemma, I said to Enid that I would return and collect her after the AA man had departed, but as I moved off, he shouted after me saying 'Ain't she with you?' It was obvious whose side he was on so we loaded up and drove away. The AC did Basingstoke and back to Bushey with driver and passenger without another murmur – truly happy days.

In 1952 we booked a joint holiday with Enid's sister and her husband at Pontin's Camp at Weston-super-Mare – well Mud Bay to be precise, up through Kewstoke Woods from the town. Enid rode her Francis Barnett autocycle, her sister Gwen drove an Argson de luxe open trike while Roy and I both had ACs to convey all the luggage. Once on the camp it seemed logical to park the bike and the Argson and make full use of the ACs with their illicit passenger carrying capacities, but this was to lead to a few exciting moments in the following couple of weeks that were to add greatly to our experience.

When driving with a passenger it was standard practice to keep an eye open for policemen, particularly if you were driving with the hood down, which made the AC a most pleasant vehicle to ride in and one of our first forays was a quick tour of Bristol for some odd reason. Heading out of the town we came upon the Avon gorge and trundled along the riverside road with Roy a good many yards ahead. As he turned on to one of the river bridges, we observed a policeman upon that bridge and just as I turned on to the bridge, the constable stepped into the roadway holding up his hand for Roy to stop. I made a hasty 'U' turn around the road island and headed out of Bristol with all the speed the AC could provide, to eventually pause in a lay-by halfway to Weston-super-Mare. After a long pause Roy came along and related the interview with the policeman which concluded with the advice that,

'I will let you go this time, but if anyone else stops you,

please don't say that I let you go!'

Our longest day out took us to Dunster and Minehead mostly in the rain but with the hood and sidescreens up protection was provided from the weather and passenger carrying in the AC became a lot less obvious until on the homeward journey we passed through Bridgwater out on to the arterial road of those days and all seemed well. Roy was, as always, some distance ahead when a police car raced past us and as it overtook Roy, it pulled in sharply and four doors opened and four policemen jumped out. It was all good gangster stuff and I was looking for a side turning that was not there, so eventually drew up behind the first AC whence the police car driver came back to me and started a cross-question session on passenger carrying on a trike.

I remained polite as one must and then produced my insurance certificate issued by the Ministry of Health. The policeman's eyes lit up as he studied the document which said, 'Limitations of use – for purposes authorised by the Policyholder'.

'Who is the policyholder?' asked the officer.

'The Ministry of Health' I replied and I was asked to promise to write to the Ministry to ask them if I was allowed to do what I was doing – passenger carrying. I readily agreed to write this letter and the interview was over. We retired for a cup of tea to regain our composure before driving back to Mud Bay.

The floral clock in the Square at Weston was an attraction for Roy and his camera and so it was that he parked in the square to take a photo from the trike, when his passenger observed an approaching policeman. There was no escape as the officer lowered his head to speak to the driver.

'You do know you are facing the wrong way in a one-way street, Sir?' he said very gravely and proceeded on his way.

It was a great holiday, but rather a strain on the nerves!'

9

Victoria

Salary rates at Art Metal were very poor and work at the Wembley factory was all a bit detached from the general business of the firm and this situation led me to apply for one or two other jobs, but none of these ever led to any great joy, so that by late 1952, the financial strain was the spur to having a loud moan in the right ear at the firm and this brought forward the offer of a job in the drawing office itself in Victoria, a prospect made possible by the possession of the new AC tricycle.

The Richards wheelchair was shipped away to SW1 by the company van and one November morning I set out in the AC for the very first of my adventurous daily journeys to London, a sequence that was to last for the next twenty years and always by trike.

Passing Neasden station, the back of Willesden bus garage, Kensal Rise station, the length of Ladbroke Grove to Notting Hill into Hyde Park and down Sloane Street to park on Ebury Bridge, where two men were detailed to march out, lift me bodily out of the trike and carry me up the steps to the wheelchair, which exercise always aroused a lot of local interest and an assured audience for the evening performance.

Getting there in the morning was one thing, but returning home after 5.30 pm was another, for the dark wet nights of November are not the best time to experiment with diversions and detours to the normal route in an effort to make better time, but worse was in store, for after only two weeks of this journey, the AC entered the workshop for repair and I was back on the Argson for my daily trip to

84

work. The rigours of 'Argson' travel are not to be envied and
on my first bracing December morning, I arrived in Hyde
Park and drove along through the frost covered grass and
trees and on to the Serpentine Bridge, where all the ducks
could be seen skating on the ice that had formed across the
width and length of the Serps. A really chilling experience
that enhanced the appreciation I always had for the protection and comfort of the AC.

The stories of incidents with the original AC and subsequently issued trikes are too numerous to recall, but typical
among them with the original trike, was blowing the water
out of the distributor with a bicycle pump.

How bleak seemed the prospects of a successful journey
home in the early 1950s before the Clean Air Act had been
established and a dense pea soup fog built up near the river
on a dark November night. Traffic built up all over London
and was even worse in the suburbs as commuters made for
home, sustenance and warmth. Temperatures were very low
and breath froze inside the windscreen as grime settled on
the outside before the days of glycerine aerosol sprays and
windscreen washers, just to add to the problems of vision
ahead. Eleven miles or so took nearly three hours that night
and if all the laws of the land had been obeyed and due
courtesy displayed to others, I would not have made it then.
The intersection at the Harrow Road and A406 junction, a
simple crossroads then, had a stationary line of traffic back up
the Harrow Road to Harlesden and the resultant jam allowed
little traffic to come in the opposite direction. The temperature in the trike, with a rug to cover my legs but no heating at
all, was by now becoming a very serious concern to me, so it
was off with the nearside sidescreen, head over the door for a
slightly better view ahead and a sight of the rear lights in front
of me and then to pull out to make a third line of traffic and
overtake the double line of stationary cars right down to the
junction at Stonebridge. This operation took a considerable
time in the filthy murky fog, but once at Stonebridge, I
managed to cross the A406 and eventually got home, frozen
to the bone and very tired, but at least the old go-kart kept
going despite the conditions of such slow travel.

On another winter's evening when an intense frost had
held all day, it was beyond my powers to get life out of the

old side-valve after standing on Ebury Bridge all day in below freezing temperatures. The lads pushed me down the hill and around the corner, but to no avail – she was quite unwilling to fire and then a car driver appeared with the insistent offer of a towed start. He towed on down to Chelsea Bridge and she did eventually burst into song, whereupon I was cast off the tow and with hasty thanks I headed for home, but all was not well, so I drew up in Sloane Street.

The brake handle on 'Model 43' had a reluctance to move far enough to apply the brakes effectively and my first thought was that ice had formed in the cable casings between the cross shaft and the rear brake drums so I gave a hefty yank on the big lever and to my horror both brake levers, one each side of the seat, rose easily from horizontal to near vertical. Both cables had frayed and my zeal had completed the severence and there we were in Sloane Street without service brake or hand brake and the temperature was still falling. Delay in getting away from Ebury Bridge had let the real rush hour go by and traffic was now lighter, all Ministry repairers would be shut and the AA could hardly be expected to solve this one in a hurry – and it was perishing cold, so I thought I would try my hand at driving completely on the engine as the gate change on the gearbox led you straight back to reverse gear that should, with luck, halt forward progress.

I always drove to some extent on the gearbox and seldom completely on the brakes, so I did have some practice in hand and this practice proved invaluable, as I made steady and very wary progress towards home. As Wembley drew near I was beginning to feel almost confident that gearboxes were made to be used in this manner providing they are backed up by an engine giving sufficient compression for braking energy.

Other odd breakdowns of lesser intensity, that served only to halt forward progress, led me, on one occasion into a sweet shop in Kilburn Lane to phone for help and on another into the Panzer delicatessen in Notting Hill Broadway, where I was thoughtfully offered a copy of that morning's *Daily Telegraph* to read while I awaited the arrival of the Ministry repairer.

Another serious incident occurred in Bayswater Road one

spring morning when the AA were summoned and duly arrived to inspect the damage and immediately departed with the Land Rover to return some time later towing a large trailer on to which the stricken trike was winched. It was rather difficult climbing up to seat level in the front of the Land Rover, but with help I made it and after washing his hands in the petrol tank underneath the driver's seat, for which purpose a sort of saucepan lid was fitted to the tank, the AA patrolman climbed abroad and we were off. All this was long before the days of 'Relay' and other such car recovery schemes, but I was impressed with the very solid feeling of the Land Rover itself as we headed out of town, although the action of the trailer was much less desirable for it was rather loosely coupled on a lynch pin and shunted to and fro in a most discomforting manner all the time.

Arriving in Kenton, the whole outfit was duly reversed into the alley behind the shops where Jim Palmer and his one employee, Joe, stood wide eyed in amazement at the new arrival. The trike was unloaded, the AA man departed and Jim took me home in the little Bradford van that served the firm so well for so many years.

The interest in the daily journeys was immense and far outweighed the problems of traffic and breakdowns. Getting to know the dingy little back streets around Ladbroke Grove as ways around a particular jam up were usually learned from trailing a knowledgeable cab driver until I was back within sight of the required route and much the same was true of the maze of side streets on the north side of the Bayswater Road, but to follow a cab here meant that he was probably heading for American settlements and clubs in the area to collect or drop a fare.

The morning trundle round Hyde Park from Lancaster Gate was always a joy, for the numbers of horses out for exercise from Knightsbridge Barracks were many and at the right season the west end of Rotten Row would be the stage for rehearsals of the musical ride by the household cavalry. The early sessions had the riders dressed in sombre khaki uniforms and as the time passed and perfection came nearer, we had full dress rehearsals with breast plates and helmets glistening in the sunshine. Eventually it would all be done to music in a less ceremonial manner with the bandsmen sitting on folding chairs beside the arena.

It was possible then to obtain a pass from the Ministry of Works, the custodian body of the Royal Parks and this would authorise you to drive a trike at not more than four miles per hour on the main pathways of the parks. This was a very useful and extremely pleasant arrangement in the mornings, for on sight of the traffic jamming up in the Bayswater Road, I could turn into Kensington Gardens opposite the Coburg Hotel and meander along the driveways to leave the gardens by the restaurant that is now an art gallery.

There were never too many people about and most of those were dog walkers whose charges ranged in size from the Irish Wolfhound to the Jack Russell Terrier and it was one of these diminutive hairy creatures that let loose from his lead, saw fit to take a great dislike to the trike one morning. The dog made very loud doggy noises as he tore around in ever diminishing circles in an arc about the trike at its statutory four mph. Eventually I was compelled to stop for fear of running the wretched thing over as its orbit got so close to the wheels. A moment later an elderly lady came galloping up, right on her last gasp and begged of the animal 'Come away, Fifi, you naughty doggy!' which the dog eventually did and I was able to continue my perambulations through the beautiful expanse of Kensington Gardens.

On one or two evenings in the years after the construction of the Hyde Park Corner underpass, the traffic from there to Marble Arch would be a six-abreast jam from which the cabbies would escape by driving down and through the underground car park escaping into North Carriage Road, but I could do even better with my pass to allay any funny looks. Down the 'No Entry' road towards the Serpentine and then turn right on to one of the main walkways leading directly up towards Lancaster Gate.

Life in the drawing office was quite hilarious at times with the strange selection of staff who came and left at intervals over the years and it was soon after my arrival at Victoria that the junior came round to my board and imparted some hushed information.

'Charlie is doing an interview,' he said, Charlie being the self-styled Chief Engineer with the unlikely christian names of Archibald Jonathan Selby – A.J.S. – a bit of a dandy with suede shoes, bow tie, camel coat, brolly, pork-pie hat and a strong thirst that always made him argumentative. A few minutes later the lad arrived again, with more tit-bits of news.

'He's interviewing a "Jerry", a German bloke,' he said and the office settled to discuss the consequences.

When he arrived to start work, the interviewee was introduced as Robert, but some wag found out that his second name was Otto, much to the annoyance of Bob who had a rather belligerent manner that did not endear him to many of his new associates. Poor old Bob tried hard to gain popularity but somehow it eluded him and his one master stroke in this attempt came a couple of years later when the Social and Sports Club of the firm was arranging the annual Christmas Party for the children of employees. A few days before the party the three boys in the drawing office were asked if they would sacrifice their Saturday to help with balloon blowing, table setting and the rest, in the hall, this being in the day when sixteen year olds were still more interested in food than in sex, since 'all the food you can eat' had been promised.

The original information about Bob had been imparted by Jack who was the eldest of the three boys and it was Jack that picked up the next gem of news to convey to my ears.

'Have you heard the latest?' he said, 'Otto has volunteered to be Father Christmas at the party. Oh, boy, we can't miss this!'

On Friday evening I bid them good night, wished them well with the party next day and went home to forget Art Metal for the weekend. I rolled in on Monday morning and retired to seclusion behind my board when Jack came round for his morning chat.

'How did the party go?' I enquired and Jack related the great time they had all had becoming caught up in the enthusiasm of the children for a really great party. 'How about Santa Claus?' I ventured.

Jack cast his eye across the office to the far corner where Bob was studying his *Daily Mirror* spread out on the board before him and then lowered his voice to tell me that, 'Otto's Santa Claus act was wonderful, marvellous and even fantastic!' I raised my eyebrows and made to enquire further but

Jack continued by saying, 'All the little boys got a pair of jack boots and all the little girls had a toy gas chamber.' Such was the attitude of teenagers in that post-war era, that I am still left to wonder what really happened.

One of the first people to meet me when I arrived in Victoria was a little man with grey hair, horn rimmed spectacles and a pipe. This was Harold who had suffered bomb damage when buried under his house in Romford, which led to a lengthy stay in hospital. All this had an adverse affect upon him and his yen to grow his own tobacco really did not help his health either, but his one intriguing ability was to be ambidextrous. It was fascinating to watch him carefully inscribe the large title across the bottom of a drawing with his left hand and mid way change to his right hand without a trace of change in the style of the lettering.

Harold's real interest was the horses and each morning he came into the office with his newspaper under his arm and so often he would pat that newspaper and say to me,

'The *Telegraph*, that's the paper for the racing.'

This led him to a handsome win on 'Never say Die' in the Derby and ever after when he was heard moaning about the work in the office, the lads would say cheerfully to him, 'Never say die, Harold!'

It was one lunchtime that Harold and I were the only two left in the office and Harold had his paper spread out over his drawing board when he burst out laughing,

'Come and read this' he said and I trundled over to his board and my eye was directed to a report of a court case of the time. It was the initial appearance of a suspect in a murder enquiry and when charged the prisoner pleaded not guilty. The arresting officer related how he had chased the suspect before apprehending him and the prisoner declared that it could not be him because he could not run.

Enquiring into this strange statement, the magistrate was told by the prisoner that he had been nobbled by the Tibbs gang.

'What did they do?' asked the magistrate and the reported reply brought tears to Harold's eyes. 'They put a shot gun down the front of my trousers', said the man, 'and they pulled the trigger.'

It was at this time that many of the drawing office staff

would be working overtime, staying three nights a week until 7.30 pm with plenty of quotations and detailing to be done. It was customary for Ron to come round in the afternoon and say 'You will stay tonight, won't you?' and this situation continued until the day I talked to Ron about a mortgage for a bungalow and asked if he would certify that I was in regular employ. We discussed home prices as Ron himself was just then taking on a house in Southall and from the conversation it transpired that my bungalow was costing £500 more than his house – and he was then the Chief Engineer! The effect was quite strange for never again was I asked to put in any overtime in that office.

For many years the printing machine in the office was a long pre–war carbon arc unit with a plate glass cylindrical drum through which the arc light could be lowered on a cable with a crude speed control gadget attached. Drawings and sensitised paper were wrapped around the drum and canvas covers drawn tight down over the paper, a process achieved with the use of a large spanner applied to the key points. The loose spanner was the cause of numerous mishaps when the print room boy would drop the spanner through one of the plate glass panels that formed the cylinder.

Access to public buildings was becoming a crusade with many disabled organisations and while I remained in employment at Victoria just such an example of this problem came up.

Brian was an associate of mine in the partitioning business at the firm and was a man of somewhat forceful character despite his interests in the Scout Association and the work he did for them. At this time the company exhibited regularly at Olympia in the Business Efficiency Exhibition and drawing office staff took turns to visit the display in order to inspect closely any new products being shown on the stands of our competitors – a sort of low level industrial espionage exercise – as well as the excuse for an afternoon out and an early night home.

When Brian suggested that it was time that I went to Olympia to see what was going on, he also offered to meet me there and push me round the exhibition, a thought to which I readily agreed and so it was that we arrived at the entrance opposite Olympia station. The steps were the first problem and Brian went inside to enquire of a level entry, which enquiry brought forth a gaily decorated member of the Royal Corps of Commissionaires. This worthy looked down at me as if I were a bad smell under his nose and proceeded to recite in parrot like tones, the wording of the official regulations, 'No hand carts, no perambulators, no dogs' he said emphatically, which caused my spirits to fall but brought forth the loud retort from Brian, 'He's not a bloody dog!'

The Commissionaire retreated hastily and brought out his superior who had a few extra layers of adornment about his person, but this worthy only endorsed the earlier remarks and there we were at the foot of the steps seemingly barred from entry to a public exhibition.

But Brian was in true fighting mood as he elbowed these two dignified specimens aside and marched straight into the hall to emerge a few minutes later with Dave, a large heavyweight Rugby player who was managing the Art Metal stand at the exhibition. Dave grabbed the chair and we marched up the road to a small door which he threw open and we were inside Olympia. This large anteroom contained some two dozen policemen, all sitting down drinking cups of tea, an occupation which ceased as we appeared and they all gazed at us with a mystified air. Across the room, through another door and we were there inside the exhibition despite the frustrating efforts of authority on that occasion.

Working at my board one afternoon, I was aware of someone standing beside me and I turned to confront a short, stout, balding man, whom I immediately offered to assist. He wanted an office built at his premises in Fulham and I produced the basic information on our product with a price guide and typical photographs, when turning further to my left, there stood another short, stout, balding man, clearly an identical twin to the first.

They were John and James, running a hire firm for chauffeur driven limousines in Farm Lane. Having satisfied their enquiry and made a date for a site survey, they departed and I returned to my work.

The next interruption came within the hour, when our door keeper, an effeminate Scotsman, arrived and said,

'Who were those chappies?' When duly informed he offered further explanation of his enquiry. The twins arrived in a chauffeur driven car – of course – but when they went downstairs, they found their chauffeur asleep, so walked up Buckingham Palace Road, hailed a cab and returned to Fulham, from where they phoned our door keeper, instructing him to wake their driver and send him home to Fulham!

In the late 1960s an elderly gentleman joined the staff to work out his last few years to retirement. His name was Basil, a long time bachelor who had only recently married; an emaciated and nervous character who nonetheless had a sense of humour and it was he who opened his eyes wide on the day I said to him

'Come on, Basil, you've been taken short!'

He blindly trailed behind, as I led the way out to the toilets at the back of the building where I threw open the casement window and drew Basil's attention to the beautiful morning outside the confines of the factory.

My timing was just right, for moments later the Royal Train drew out of the near platforms of Victoria station with its significant headcode. Basil did not believe it was the Royal Train although it was Derby Day and he knew the Queen would be going to Epsom for the occasion, but his disbelief turned to great excitement as the open royal saloon came under the lavatory window and there, sitting on the facing longitudinal seat, was quite unmistakably, the Queen herself with another lady as companion.

The process of viewing special trains from that window was not too difficult as the newspapers gave times of street closures in Victoria and an approximation of the arrival of the procession from Buckingham Palace either for the departure of the Queen or her guest or the arrival of a State visit by a foreign dignatory. Thus it was that I saw the arrival of the trains carrying the President of France, the Shah of Persia and the Emperor of Japan en route from Gatwick Airport.

It was also possible to have a regular view of the electric Brighton Belle Pullman, right there under the window or on the far side continental tracks, the Wagons Lit Blue Train and the Golden Arrow, hauled successively by the Bulleid *Merchant Navy*, the BR Standard Pacifics, notably *William Shakespeare* and latterly by the Southern Electric locomotives.

In the 1950s steam was still well visible at Victoria and

right under our window was the turntable where it was a regular sight to see one of the Marsh Atlantics, *Trevose Head, St Alban's Head* or the like being turned round for their next journey to Oxted and to watch the strenuous efforts of the footplate men as they struggled to get the great turntable moving with the locomotive carefully positioned to get the balance right for turning.

Plate layers often worked under this window with a huge hacksaw in a frame, clamped to a piece of railway line to which a heavy weight was fixed to the outer end of the saw and a vertical lever to the near end, so that two men could push this lever to and fro in a rowing action to cause the hacksaw to move backwards and forwards over the rail to very gradually cut through this one hundredweight per yard section of high quality steel.

I never had time to see a full cut made in this manner, but the other interesting performance below the window was the pile of firewood and loco coal used to raise a rail section to red heat – after a time – when the rail could be lowered into another gee clamp in the centre of which a heavy screw thread would press on the side of the rail, while two men leaned mightily upon a six foot tommy-bar to advance the screw and so gradually bend the red hot rail – and this was outside Victoria station in the 1950s!

Such were the delights of Victoria before total electrification ended it all.

10

Matrimony

The ups and downs of driving around 'two-up' in the brown AC led eventually to the engagement of myself to Enid Mary Taylor and arrangements for marriage were planned. We decided to invest in a motorcar while keeping the AC and passing Enid's Francis Barnet autocycle over to her father for those early morning trips to Garston bus garage.

A lot of cars were viewed in a lot of different places until we decided to purchase a 1939 Series 'E' Morris 8 with rear hinged doors which gave some advantage in falling backwards into the car from a standing position with the legs and hips locked out straight. Reselco hand control gear was fitted for £39. 10s. and the car was delivered into the sideway of 78 Barnhill Road, where my first effort at driving a car was to reverse it out, uphill along the long driveway of the house and out into the road.

My father was persuaded to renew the driving licence that he held in 1931–2 before the days of the driving test and Enid's father likewise, so that we had two licensed drivers to accompany us on our trial runs prior to the driving test at Hendon, where the examiner kindly agreed to a pass certificate and we were away!

The wedding was at the Congregational Church in Wembley Park, attended by all members of both families with the exception of Cyril and Dorothy Porter for the sad reason that Cyril's mother died that very morning. A lot of ITA folk were there as the photographs show and after the ceremony we set off in the Morris 8 for our first long drive in the direction of the Lake District.

St Albans and the A6 to Loughborough for a one night stay

in a hotel and then on via Derby, Sheffield, Salford, Manchester, Preston, Lancaster, Carnforth and Kendal to Ambleside and up the Langdale Valley to a very pleasant hotel where the ground floor annexe was an old Lakeland gun powder factory. An excellent, if rather damp, honeymoon was spent in Langdale and the only snag with the Morris was the ascent of Shap Fell on the old A6 in the pouring rain when a yellow duster became entangled in the complicated mechanical drive of the solitary windscreen wiper which promptly ceased to operate. Driving over Shap Fell in this weather without a wiper, however puny, was a difficult experience, but once down into Penrith, salvation was to hand at the expense of a new wiper motor.

We had trips up to Keswick as well as Windermere and the nearer lakes and to the west over Wrynose Pass to Wrynose Bottom, but not daring to take the Morris 8 on the steeper slopes of Hard Knott, we pressed on southwards through Ulverston and along the coast to Ravensglass for a quick look at the Ravensglass and Eskdale Railway.

Our first major trip over, it was back to Barnhill Road and the weary grind to Victoria every day, while Enid travelled to Watford to maintain her job at the Gas Board there. For long the AC did the length of Barnhill Road every morning with Enid as passenger on her way to Wembley Park station, but the sad day came when some busybody informed the Ministry of Health of my illicit passenger carrying and a sharp note arrived from Woodgrange House threatening to withdraw the AC. The value of the trike to us was untold and so the morning trips had to be abandoned probably to the delight of that prying eye, who never did identify himself. Life went on while we saved very hard for the future, living in the downstairs front room of Barnhill Road.

The old car continued to perform well, if somewhat lethargically, with a top speed never above 50 mph, but returning a creditable 45 mpg which was nearly as good as the trike. There were regular visits to Baughhurst with Enid and my mother in the back and my father in front with me, trundling down the Bath Road to Aldermaston and as we always went on Good Friday, it would coincide with the 'Ban the Bomb' Easter march from the AWRE at Aldermaston to Trafalgar Square for a big demonstration of anti nuclear protest. The long straggling column was always a motley collection of intellectual and society drop-outs, all of dishevelled appearance.

In 1955 we booked ourselves into a boarding house in Torquay for the holiday but this was only a partial success as I was expected to be seated in the dining room before everyone else arrived in order to allay disturbance of the other guests and the ground floor lavatory was in the hallway with a queue each morning, all aggravated by the fact that I could not manage to lock the door on the inside after being helped down on the seat, so Enid had to do sentry-go outside the door. The photos in the dining room were all of Salvation Army bands which conveyed little to me until I met the proprietor coming in the front gate on a Sunday evening carrying his euphonium on his uniformed arm.

Marriage to Enid, apart from the basic joys, was probably the most emphatic encouragement to independence in my life, as it added the spur to launch into activities that earlier parental influence had always been afraid to encourage. Much of this is explained in the surrounding chapters, but having a sister with polio brought Enid wide experience of dealing with the myriad problems that constantly present themselves in these circumstances.

Enid was the eldest of three children in the Taylor family and was three years older than myself. Brought up in Bushey, she was a very studious pupil at school and took life seriously, joining the 5th Bushey Girl Guides, from where her eventual reputation for organising ability probably stems. From a place at Watford Grammar School she achieved a good School Certificate with seven credits. This and her flair for maths led to her attendance for interview at Radiant House, the headquarters of the Watford and St Albans Gas Company early in the war.

The interview was conducted by one William Evetts, an awesome man who was then Production Engineer of the company, a surviving officer from the Somme over which he often reminisced and now the commander-in-chief of three coal gas plants and wide distribution network. Taylor finances were limited, so that when she appeared for that interview, which was to affect her life for the next thirty years, she was still dressed in her school gymslip, a story that was oft repeated by her boss in later years, to her great embarrassment!

Radiant House was the pinnacle of gas company policy, the entire building being still lit by gas in the 1940s. Work in the small drawing/stats office was exacting and thorough including such mundane work as the collation of daily, weekly, monthly etc production and output figures to the more exciting calculation of paint quantities for the camouflage of gas holders! This work eventually led to evening classes at Watford Technical College, then in Queens Road, Watford, and after three years, to success in the examinations for an Ordinary National Certificate in Mechanical Engineering at a high standard. Thus armed and inspired she then went on to Willesden Technical College at the time of the doodlebugs, in an effort to achieve a Higher National Certificate in this subject. However, the strains of wartime living and home problems, combined with her work at the local Congregational Church proved too much and following a breakdown, she abandoned these academic pursuits temporarily, but for various reasons they were never resumed.

Although she had a fleeting interest in joining the WRNS, this was thwarted by the interests of the gas company, when her position was declared 'technical assistant' and it became a reserved occupation, an action which probably made this story possible!

11

Scotland

On that holiday in Torquay we conducted one or two experiments with a little 'Woolworth' spirit stove – a very crude but effective means of boiling a kettle with methylated spirits burning fiercely. It was this trial that really got us under way with grand plans for 1956, which were so successful that we truly had the holiday of our lifetime in Scotland.

The first item purchased was a bright shining brass Optimus pressure stove, to have the burner heated with 'meth' before pumping the base container up to a pressure that fed a minute jet of paraffin through the hot burner hole to ignite and roar away for an hour or more so that a whole cooking process could be achieved by careful manipulation of the sequence of operations. Hot water for tea, shaving, washing and washing up, as well as milk to fill vacuum flasks, the frying of egg, bacon, tomato and bread, all arranged to arrive more or less when required.

A selection of billy cans was purchased along with sleeping bags and a canvas bed on steel rods that could be opened out and sprung into place, but in folded form was no more than three feet long and a few inches in diameter. A good groundsheet came next and a selection of square biscuit tins into which all the household items, the stove and fuel could be packed neatly away.

Summoning all the experience of a life with the Girl Guide movement and using all the instruction that could be gathered from that source, egged on by brief experience of making tea on the Woolworth's meth burner, we began to plan the more adventurous holiday for 1956.

A six foot six inch ridge tent was borrowed from the Bushey Guides and a trial pitching performed in the garden to ensure that it was quite possible for the two of us to erect a ridge tent without further aid. The process was to lay the tent out flat to one side of the centre line of erection, feed the three ridge poles through the canvas and fit the finials and main guy ropes thereto. Bang in the four corner pegs, hitch two guy ropes on one side of these pegs and then with one of us at each end, we could lift the main poles and the canvas to the vertical, whence Enid could hitch on the second rope at her end and adjust them both up to stand firm and then come to anchor my end of the tent, after which the walls could be pegged down, the ground sheet laid and all the junk of camping moved inside.

With the Morris 8 now seventeen years old, we loaded the tent, groundsheet, folding beds, sleeping bags, biscuit tins full of provisions and toiletries and the Optimus pressure paraffin stove with a supply of paraffin and methylated spirit, a suitcase full of clothes, a couple of cushions and the wheelchair. The back seat cushion was removed and the rear compartment scientifically loaded in a sequence of possible necessity and then the rear boot was filled in a similar manner before we bolted the bar between the brackets on the back bumper that served as a carrier for the wheelchair and was an adaptation of the wheelchair carrier that I had made some years before to fix this same wheelchair on to the side of the footwell of my open Argson tricycle. With a three miles to the inch mapbook and a large white AA map of England and Scotland on which our proposed route was marked out in red pencil, we were ready to set out on a Saturday morning. Our finances were £35 in cash, a cheque book, a good supply of sweets and a pair of crutches. When the Morris was capable of 45 miles per gallon, it was not surprising that not much over 45 miles per hour was possible, so progress before the days of the Motorway was not sensational. However, an early start from Wembley got us into the Lake District.

That Saturday evening we arrived at Kendall and found our way to Sampool Farm where we were directed to the camping field by a lady who told us joyfully that the toilets were 'over there in the hedge, but they are not very nice', which was hardly an encouraging start to my camping experience. We set up the tent, all as our practice run and the paraffin stove was soon under way to cook the meal and make tea as well as fill a flask for a late night drink to make the most economical use of the stove while it was going. It was a tiring day and we climbed into our sleeping bags which to me were surprisingly warm and snug and I was soon fast asleep, although somewhat conscious of the vulnerability of that thin sheet of canvas between me and the outside world.

I slept very well, but came to quite suddenly in the dark hours to hear the rain belting down on the tent and wonder of wonders, it did not come through! I listened for a moment and became aware of another strange sound that was uncomfortably close to my ear that in turn was uncomfortably close to the ground, from which this munching and rending noise was coming. Cows had been let into the field and were tearing the grass from the ground around the tent with not a thought for the torrents of rain that were bucketing down on to the tent canvas. This together with the proposition in the hedge, was life at its rural worst and I began to have doubts about the wisdom of camping. Sunday morning however, dawned bright and clear and the night-time thoughts were soon forgotten as we manoeuvred around the ablutionating problems, dressed including the time-consuming assembly of the mechanical man around me and made breakfast of cereal and milk, followed by egg, bacon, tomato and fried bread, all processed on the stove, which it fell to my lot to operate as well as assembling and packing away in the biscuit tin after use.

Then back on to the A6, northwards over Shap Fell, the Morris chugging along under its considerable load without too much sign of strain, onward through Carlisle and over the border into real Scotland for the first time in our lives. A brief pause was made in Gretna Green out of curiosity before searching the town of Dumfries for the camp site attached to a garage on the far side. Here was a beautiful clean site with close mown grass and a water closet on the garage that was quite easy to enter straight from the wheelchair. Camping suddenly seemed to be that much more attractive as the evening sunshine shimmered through the heat rising from the pressure stove where an evening meal was being cooked, by the scientific process of switching pots and pans in the necessary sequence to bring each item on the menu to the 'table' more or less at the appropriate time and culminating with the washing up water before most items were packed away again for the morning chores next day.

That beautiful accessible toilet was a great joy next morning and the feeding, washing and packing process was completed with a little more precision so that we were soon on the road across the lowlands, heading for the coast at Ayr and following the coast road northwards to Wemyss Bay where we turned into a quite magnificent caravan park set on a wooded hillside overlooking the sea. It looked very grand and far away above our humble tent, but our prior correspondence had agreed we could pitch here, so equipped with this letter, Enid approached the caravan to end all caravans, where the site owner was sitting proudly in the most advantageous position on the site. Of the conversation, I caught but little, but what I did catch included '. . . my husband's got a wheelchair . . . Oh, my dear, you must park here, it will be just right for you. . .' And just right it was, on the large close cropped lawn in front of that caravan to end all caravans with an uninterrupted view across miles of open sea towards Rothesay. The toilets were in a block house that was only reasonably accessible but we managed and the weather remained fine and dry, so our view of camping was gaining enthusiasm.

Waking next morning not too long after sunrise, I pushed back the tent flap and lay there near to the ground; the view was tremendous as the early morning sun shone out there on misty Bute and the first boat of the day was sailing away from Wemyss pier that was only just visible under the hillside. This was certainly the life, despite the toilet block and the morning routine was entered into with great expectations for the day ahead, that was not to disappoint us.

Camp struck and the Morris loaded, we continued northward along the banks of the Clyde through the ship building area with those massive cranes towering every-where, up as far as the Erskine Ferry where we had a lengthy wait even as ferries go and we had time to ponder on our day's programme. Once our turn came to board the ferry boat, we were soon out on the Dumbarton shore and heading for the bonny banks of Loch Lomond. Our first sight of a

Scottish loch was everything we had read about as we wound our way along the main road as far as Tarbet before turning westward away from the Loch and towards Arrochar where the road divides for 'Rest and be Thankful', the old RAC hill climb, now circumnavigated by a long straight main road, that climbed on a steady gradient to the brow of the hill before turning the corner and sweeping down toward Loch Fyne whose shore we followed round the end of the loch and back to Inverary passing the castle on the way. Northwards we went under the arch in the town and to Dalmally on the main road to the west through the Pass of Brander and along the banks of Loch Awe. This was quite a hard day's drive with the Morris and constant nudging and pinching of the mechanical man ensured that I did not fall asleep as we trundled along in glorious Argyllshire. A few miles before Oban, we came to Connel Ferry Bridge where the railway line to Ballachulish spanned Loch Etive and we joined the small queue for our turn to drive over the sleeper bed beside the single railway line, on payment of four shillings toll to British Rail.

This charge seemed rather high at the time and caused me to wonder what the charge would be for the vehicle following behind us. This was a large Austin Sheerline and hitched on the back was a stately caravan like a thatched cottage on wheels and pro rata to the Morris 8, it should have been charged a princely sum in tolls on the Connel Bridge.

This impressive steel girder bridge led us to Benderloch and Rubbarb Farm where camping facilities were said to exist. The smell of farmyard was everywhere and the ground was mown stalks of some crop or other, while the water supply was from a tap in the cowshed along with the cows, which Enid was not very keen on visiting. However, it had been a hard day and we decided to make the best of it as we set up the tent for as reasonable a night as the affluvia would allow.

Next morning we left the tent where it stood and went down into Oban town to walk along the sea front, watch the MacBrayne steamer, take a look in the Scottish shops and then climb Pulpit Hill, a high vantage point to the south west of the town where the park benches offered a tremendous panorama over the length of the seafront right up through the town to McCaig's Tower standing like an unfinished cake on the hillside. The weather was grand and the comparative peace of this tourist resort where the steamer was loading one or two cars for shipment to the islands, was a true delight.

Reluctantly we drove out of the town for another four bobs' worth on the bridge and back to Rubbarb Farm where we decided to pack up the tent as the stiff stalks under the groundsheet were a great hazard and move across the road to the common land opposite the farm where better ground was to be found. We filled the water carrier at the farm tap to see us over our morning ablutions, but the toilet situation was much as we had experienced on our first night's camping – somewhat difficult.

Packing up next day, assembling the mechanical man, who thankfully had shown no signs of breakage despite the many contortions I had to perform to get in and out of the car, down to the ground from the wheelchair and back again, which was even more strenuous. This last manoeuvre was necessitated by my domestic chores of controlling the pressure stove, some elementary supervision of the cooking and the washing up which were all dealt with at ground level, so that nothing could fall anywhere and in any case we had no room to carry a table with the load already on the Morris 8.

Northwards from Benderloch and goodbye to Rubbarb Farm, we followed the railway line as it wound its way up to the ferry at Ballachulish before we wandered on to Kinloch-leven past the big terminus in the village. The occasional train was hauled by an ex Caledonian tank engine approaching its own twilight years along with those of the branch line itself. Queueing for the ferry boat was a tedious business that we omitted, reaching North Ballachulish by the longer route around Loch Leven and then along the coast road to Fort William, the base town for Ben Nevis adventurers. On the approach to the town facing Loch Linnhe were a long line of bungalows and each had a fair acreage of ground attached most of which was let over to camping sites which were almost vying with each other for business. Our selected and pre-arranged spot loomed up and we drove into a very nice, although somewhat crowded site, complete with all mod cons and a pleasant night was spent within site of Loch

Linnhe.

The weather held up next morning and we strolled along Fort William High Street to view the shops, but alas we did not inspect the railway station then in its last years with steam locomotives. Out of Fort William towards Spean Bridge and The Great Glen with its cattle ranch, on to Fort Augustus and a first sight of Loch Ness, the Morris 8 chugging along seemingly quite happy as we took the west shore main road past Urquart Castle and eventually into Inverness.

In 1956, the old road bridge still stood spanning the shallow waters of the River Ness, a bridge with towers at the town end and suspension cables out across the span. Over the bridge, through the main street and out on to the main A9 as it wound its way up the several miles of climb to the Cairngorm area. Some three miles up the hill was Inshes camping ground, a bungalow of some age, sideways on to the road, with tent camping on the up side and caravan parking lower down. We moved in, set up the tent and all the gear, had a quick inspection of the log cabin toilet, interviewed the old boy in the bungalow and paid our half crown for each of a two night stay. The one enduring memory of Inshes site in the dusk is the procession of lorries that ground their way so noisily up the long incline from Inverness all loaded with Coran's kippers!

Next day we spent in Inverness, a very nice little town, capital of the Highlands as it claims to be, with its very Scottish shops and its market arcade where every permanent stall bore a really local name – except one. A jewellers and watchmakers advertising sight testing and painless ear piercing was under the very un-Scottish name of 'Finklestien'.

We had an excellent lunch in a restaurant on the far side of the river close to the bridge, where four years later an evening was spent down on Ness Side by the water, when the wail of bagpipes drifted in across the way. Then we strolled on up river to the foot bridge, crossed over to bring the sounds nearer and followed on to the Northern Meeting Ground, a sort of cricket field with a large covered pavilion for admittance to which we were charged a modest sum. Once inside, it was Highland Night for visitors. The British Legion Pipe Band, a local school of dancing where the tiny kilt clad girls performed Highland Flings and much else before a young lady appeared on the trailer stage in the middle of the ground to sing sweet Scottish songs like the *Northern Lights of Auld Aberdeen* followed by a kilted 'he-man' in a Harris tweed jacket with a dagger in his socks, who sang unaccompanied songs in Gaelic – a most extraordinary performance.

This was also the day the Morris 8 gave a bit of trouble as the brake could be pressed continually forward with little or no effect on progress. A large garage adjacent to the railway station was visited and the sole help there was the offer to sell us a new complete master cylinder, but what good would that be without the fitting? We retreated to see the AA man at the entrance to the town. He looked saddened and told us the bad news that it was 'Trades Week', a sort of Scottish 'Wakes Week' and everyone would be closed for business and then he brightened up and suggested an agricultural engineer just up the road – 'Go and see him and tell him I sent you!' Following this advice, we had the ready fitting of two new washers in the master cylinder and a refill of brake fluid, all for thirty-five shillings.

The next morning, with all gear packed aboard, we headed south on the old A9 to Carrbridge and took the road up to Grantown on Spey, a very clean and pleasant place on the edge of Grant Castle grounds, along the A939 and so onward to Tomintoul, the highest village in Britain and rather forlorn and bleak. After this the A939 dwindled to a sort of cart track with two tarmac covered wheel ruts and a high grass ridge down the centre. Passing places were really essential and these were all marked with long stakes carrying a small white diamond. Up on the high barren moorland, the miles of this terrain rolled by until the winding descent to the original Cock Bridge and up the steep winders on the other side.

We paused here to rest the Morris 8 as we were steadily gaining on an ex-London taxicab ahead. It appeared to be about to cough its last, when it stopped and a number of young people climbed out, which explained the problem. They all leaned hard on the back of the cab and the driver was thus able to breast the next incline before they all bundled aboard again and were off. The cab was the only sign of life for miles and we let him get a mile or two in front before following on along the rest of the A939 to Ballater and Royal Deeside.

The camp site at Ballater was most picturesque but not very well appointed. It lay well below the road down by the riverside, was void of a useable toilet and the water supply was described as a 'spring' emerging from a pipe in the banking around the site. On a later visit we took a quick look inside Craithie Church, arriving with a tourist coach party, which served to fill the pews and when the verger clapped eyes on me, he immediately uncoupled the heavy rope strung across the aisle and wheeled me out in front of the congregation before commencing his recital of historical notes. Grasping the wheelchair firmly I was pointed towards the bust of the Duke of 'so-and-so' while the dialogue was recited and then spun round to face the next item in his catalogue and so it went on, with half the visitors paying due heed to his words and the other half with their eyes glued to my unwilling gyrations before the altar.

Having escaped, we retreated for lunch to the most accessible restaurant around, which just happened to be on Ballater railway station, where a goodly meal was consumed, as I made a careful study of the assorted crockery and cutlery on the table. The vintage varied greatly with BR emblems on much of the crockery and older LNER and LMS initials on the cutlery, but the prize piece was a solitary teaspoon from the Great North of Scotland Railway that died in 1923.

In 1956 we only stayed on this primitive camp site at Ballater for one night before moving on past Balmoral to Braemar and the Devil's Elbow, as it was then and into the Spittal of Glen Shee, heading for Dundee and the Tay ferry boat service. These were sizeable boats each loading some forty cars for the 2¼ mile crossing of the River Tay with a landing in Fife where a short drive brought us into St Andrews and the cliff top camp site run by the local council. Driving the Morris in for a quick tour of the site, we set up camp on the large tent area and settled down in the sleeping bags for a good night's rest, that was shattered at a very early hour by raucus bugle calls from the Boys' Brigade camp installed close by.

Away next morning along the coast road through the tiny ports of Crail and Anstruther, till we came in sight of the Forth Bridge, one of the wonders of the Railway Age, built in the 1890s and being painted continuously ever since. North Queensferry saw us on a ferry boat again, this time not quite so large as the Tay boats, carrying only some twenty eight cars on the slightly shorter crossing of the Firth of Forth.

On the A8, a few miles west of Edinburgh, near the Royal Show Ground was a garage with a close mown field behind, let out for camping and here we settled in for a couple of nights stay. The field was excellent and suitable toilet facilities were on the island of petrol pumps on the garage forecourt. The strange thing about this was, as the door opened for the wheelchair to be brought within reach, you would find yourself sitting there looking straight down the A8 towards Glasgow and all the oncoming traffic looking at you!

The next day was spent in Edinburgh visiting the castle, walking Princes Street, then lined with Scottish shops and having lunch in one of the numerous Crawford's restaurants that were advertised as always being within five minutes walk of wherever you were in Princes Street. Back to the camp site for the night before heading for the border via Dalkeith and a one night stop at York and then home.

In fourteen days, the old Morris 8 had clocked up 1,940 miles, the only cough being the incident in Inverness. We set out with £35 in cash and a cheque book. After buying food, petrol, paying camp site charges, ferry tolls and the car repair, we came home with £7 and an unused cheque book! Surely the greatest and most economical holiday we have ever had – haste ye back and we did!

12

Carry on Camping

The experimental holiday of 1956 convinced us of the possibilities and desirabilities, not to mention the economics of camping, so we invested in a ridge pole tent of our own and began planning our excursions for 1957. Westwards to Wales, camping at Coleford on the way to Aberystwyth and then northwards to Beddgelert with the object of taking a closer look at Portmadoc and the newly reinstated Festiniog Railway.

Although trains were running across the Cob, the whole appearance was hardly likely to inspire any but the hardened enthusiast. One of the Fairlie locomotives was in steam and the stock was usable, but little more, while on the track bed the grass grew healthily and the station building was scarcely more than a shell.

We presented ourselves at the Llanberis station of the Snowdon Mountain Railway where a handful of tourists queued for seats on the next train to the summit. I approached a member of the staff and enquired of the possibilities of boarding the train myself and to my great surprise the response was 'Certainly, sir, come this way sir!' He led the way on to the platform, past the little rack locomotive with its valves lifting from a good head of steam, along the single almost toastrack coach to the front of the train, where I was lifted into the brakeman's compartment followed by the folded wheelchair and Enid, all with the brakeman himself and his big screw down brake wheel that made the tiny compartment at the front rather cramped.

The front windows gave an excellent view on to the track ahead, out over the little bridge and up on to the hillside of

109

the lower slopes of Snowdon. With the doors all shut and the whistle blown, we moved gently forward with the sound of the locomotive blowing hard, but a strange lack of any sense of power being exerted on our progress. As the nose of the coach began to rise on the first incline, the driver opened up and the real power of the loco was felt by a tremendous boost to our progress and this continued to the rapid exhaust beats all the way up to the passing loop at the halfway stage of the climb where we stopped for water. As we climbed steeply at a modest rate of knots, the brakeman gave us a private commentary on what there was to be seen to left and right and this informative discourse continued right to the Summit station where we were off-loaded on to the platform to take a brief stroll · with the wheelchair out on to the top of real Mount Snowdon.

We boarded the next train for the descent with the locomotive preceding us and lowering us very gently down the steep winding track back to Llanberis; a full hour for climbing and another full hour for the return journey, but one of the most fascinating trips I have ever made.

In 1958 we set out for Scotland, still with the Morris 8 laden with camping equipment and set up the tent at Inshes camping ground on the A9 three miles south of Inverness, where strolling round the shops in the main street we came upon a lorry delivering fresh meat to a butcher's shop. The vehicle was a large van with canvas side curtains drawn apart for the driver to lift the carcases on to his shoulder and into the shop. As he dragged one such huge piece of beastie off the van, a sheep's head came with it and fell neatly on the kerb, to be retrieved by the driver when he returned. He bent down, grabbed the sheep's head and tossed it back into the van where it fell with a plop into a sea of blood that covered the floor of the vehicle and duly splattered around both inside and outside the van.

The Morris 8 had served us well for six years, when we became more ambitious and our minds turned to a small van as these were free of purchase tax until you fitted windows in the sides.

With no real knowledge of vans and not too much about cars, we set out to visit the Commercial Motor Show at Earls Court where we hoped to see the van selection on the market, but it was not to be.

Driving the Morris around Earls Court looking for a parking place was difficult and became even more difficult when the Morris stopped dead in a side street. The law gathered round and said politely,

'You can't stop there, Sir!', but I had little option as the car refused to respond to persuasion. One constable explained carefully that if they allowed you to stay there, the residents would phone the station and they would be in trouble, but after careful assessment of the car and me, they became almost over helpful until the foreman of policemen strolled up the street and there was a brief conference, a stately nodding of heads and off he went, while the policemen and I peered under the bonnet.

There was much chiding among the officers, 'Don't let Harry touch it – his so and so motor car never works!' they said, when a gentleman escorting two ladies happened along the other side of the road. Seeing the policemen and me leaning over the car, this immaculately dressed gentleman abandoned his lady friends, crossed the road towards us and enquired of the trouble. He knew that we did not know and removed his gloves and his white scarf, handed them to a policeman, did a rapid one, two, three under the bonnet, declared it to be the SU electric pump, sorted through my limited tool roll and removed the offending pump from the bulk head of the engine compartment.

The immaculate gentleman wiped his hands on the proffered piece of rag, handed me the pump with instructions on the nearest garage to visit for help, and he was gone! While the law stood guard over the Morris, Enid pushed the chair down the road to the garage, where we had to wait the return of the breakdown wagon to acquire a trade–in pump, whence we trundled back to the car.

The policemen were obviously finding my problems more interesting than controlling the traffic and as we all mused on the fitting of the new pump, a small van tore up the road, parked just in front of us, two men jumped out and took the fitting job out of our hands.

Within ten minutes the Morris was ticking over again, the two men leapt back into their van and departed with barely a word, leaving the policemen to bid us a safe journey home and us to wonder just who the immaculate gentleman was who probably arranged our salvation that day.

In 1960, the Annual General Meeting of the ITA was at Giffnock on the outskirts of Glasgow, so we set off with our new A35 van for our first night's camp at High Heskett on the A6 and arrived in Giffnock by 10 am the next morning in time for the start of the meeting held in a large school with sleeping accommodation in the classrooms. On Sunday we set off into Scotland proper by way of Stirling on the A9 and Inverness, onward north along the east coast for a quick look at Wick and then camped in Thurso overlooking the sea with its extended hours of daylight.

Along the coast westwards to Scourie and down the far side of Sutherland with its wild and deserted beaches to Gairloch, Loch Maree, Garve and Strome Ferry, thus up and over to Kyle of Lochalsh.

While camped at Kyle, we surveyed the steamer timetables displayed at the railway station on the pier and decided that an afternoon sail from Kyle down to Mallaig would be desirable. Boats are able to tie up on all three sides of the pier, the head being equipped with re-fuelling outlets and on this day the village side of the pier was occupied by a rather scruffy trawler of some kind with a naval crew and I assumed that the steamer would berth on the pier end, but alas I was mistaken. When the McBrayne flag hove in sight, the tedious process of coming alongside eventually brought the steamer to tie up on the far side of the trawler whence the gangway was lowered to the trawler and all the passengers disembarked by trailing around the deck of the trawler and climbing another steep gangplank up to the pier.

Having surveyed this process and decided that we would not be sailing that day, the station master appeared – the railway station is right there on the pier – and enquired if I were thinking of going on the boat. 'Yes', I said, 'I was thinking but . . . ', whereupon the station master waved his arm and we were confronted by a naval officer in gold braid and epaulettes. A brief and earnest conversation in a deep Scottish tongue took place and the officer surveyed me as if I were a bad smell under his nose, before barking out those unintelligible words of command that brought two seamen to attention before him. More staccato words of command were snapped out and before I had time to protest, the seamen had hoisted me aloft and how fortunate that the chair was a Dingwall 'County' with fixed footrests as the man at the front grabbed these and his colleague took the handles behind.

With the man in front walking backwards, his face level with my knees, we progressed towards the gangplank that protruded a foot or so above the deck of the pier before descending at a steep angle. My mind was firmly fixed on that protrusion and the height I was above the decking, as my friend stepped backwards up and over the end of the gangplank and we began to descend the slatted slope with the chair held so high that the wheels were clear of the handrails of the gangway. I looked over the side and for a brief moment I could see the wet water a long way below, so I turned my eyes to the backwards walking man in front of me to see the sweat pouring down his face and over the hairs on his chest and I prayed that he would not collapse as almost the entire weight of the operation was on him. We reached the deck of the trawler and I prepared to be set down on my wheels, but that was not to be, for the sweating tars continued holding me aloft as we paraded round the trawler and eventually made our way up the next gangway to the steamer with the same man still walking backwards before me.

I was set down on the deck and the seamen vanished rapidly to what I trust was due reward but this I never discovered, but it was then that I noticed the pier rail lined with people and the steamer rail likewise all gazing at me, obviously having taken full note of my stately, if precarious progress to the safety of the deck where I now rested. The steamer crew had also seen all this and were keeping their distance from me as they had visions ot getting me back to that pier after the voyage but they need not have feared. It was a very pleasant sail down the coast to Mallaig and all its seagulls and then back to Kyle of Lochalsh where two seamen carried me and Enid took the chair on to the pier with not too much effort.

In 1963, intent on a holiday in the Emerald Isle, we set off one fairly bright morning in June along the monotonous miles of the A1 and the Great North Road to Scotch Corner and then westwards on A66 over Stainmore to Penrith. A brief skirmish around this Cumberland market town in search of food on a Saturday evening was not too rewarding and we retreated to the van with a parcel of fish and chips.

Onward along A6, we reached High Heskett for a night in the tent to sleep off those 300 miles and then awoke to a bright sunny dawn for food, ablutions and de–camping to make an early start for the border and on through Kirkcud-brightshire and Wigtown to Stranraer. It was at Stranraer that evening that it all began, that merciless, relentless, steady rain that pattered on the tent canvas and generally brought chilly damp depression all around. Praise be to the inventor of the flea bag for bringing a degree of warmth and comfortable sleep to help you forget the rain – but to no avail, for on waking at seven on Monday morning, it was still there – that rhythmic pitter–patter that meant a damp departure from the camp site.

With the morning chores behind and everything packed in the van, there was time for a look round what there is of Stranraer and a short ride to Kirkcolm in a vain hope of losing the rain, then back to the pier for the 2.30 boat.

Marine travel presents its own problems for a wheelchair, but getting aboard a car ferry is simply not among them. Prior notice of my difficulties to the port office proved quite useful, for a member of the crew came to survey the line of cars and eventually approached me with the question,

'Are you the gentleman that is encumbered?'

I had to think for a moment before I could bring myself to agree and we were then escorted straight down on to the huge car deck and parked beside a hatchway. Out of the van and into the wheelchair and there stood the fatigue party, who lifted me smartly through the hatchway and up two flights of stairs to the first class deck. There were more stairs to the second class deck, but the fatigue party fell out very smartly at first class level before the loudspeaker announced that second class passengers found on first class deck would be charged the excess fare. They did not look very hard to find the offenders before we sailed and once out in the Irish Sea, the heave-ho set in and all the best people left the first class dining room, whereupon we were invited in and seated at a secluded table for two with a reserved notice thereon.

'Would you like some tea?'

'Not 'arf–er, yes please!'

Then followed a large pot of tea, a plate of fancy cakes and an hour or so's yarn with the steward in the absence of other customers.

The one boat on the Stranraer/Larne service did two round trips a day, leaving Stranraer at 7 am for the first crossing and getting back at 9 pm from the second, six days a week, with one trip on Sundays.

With Larne coming steadily closer, I was whisked back down the stairs, through the hatchway and into the car, just in time to hear the announcement

'Will car drivers please return to their vehicles.'

With the tailboard down, the hundred-odd vehicles tore out into the quiet streets of Larne and we were in Ireland! Follow the signs to Belfast, twenty one miles and keep a look out for the promised escort on the city boundary and there they were – the trikes of Mr and Mrs Kidd to lead the way round the city streets of Belfast, along the dockyard, over the Laggan and out to 159 Ravenshill Road, Ballynafeigh House, the proud possession of the Belfast and District Group of the DDA.

On our arrival, a substantial reception committee were seated in the lounge and a 'you must be hungry' cry went up as Miss Secretary wheeled in two enormous ham salads, which we consumed with some difficulty, whilst endeavouring to keep up a conversation with all around. The hospitality and welcome by the Belfast group was something to be experienced, as was the comfort of the only ground floor bedroom with its twin beds and yellow counterpanes.

A week's stay at Ballynafeigh House produced one nice afternoon, which fortunately coincided with a drive along the Antrim coast northwards and westwards from Larne, where for twenty miles the road followed the rocky coast and ran close to the sea all the way. There were also visits to Ballymena, Ballymoney, Bangor, Downpatrick and the rest, but the rain was rather persistent, so a visit to Belfast Transport Museum was indicated. This museum, tucked away in a back street, contained a very interesting selection of locomotives, trams, a traction engine, motor cycles, push bikes, fire engines and cars of mature years, also some fine examples of horsedrawn carriages. Arriving at an off peak hour, we were treated to an unofficial conducted tour, when the workings of many of the exhibits were exclusively demonstrated. The neatly disappearing steps of the stately carriages and the modesty windows, the Minerva cab in which Churchill left Belfast at the time of the 'troubles' and the Belfast tramcar on which is displayed the notice 'the rule of the sea is women and children first' – ever been to sea in a tram?

This visit spurred us on to the other more orthodox museum with its art gallery of finely detailed landscape paintings depicting many square miles of Irish countryside with every tiny detail of cottages and hedgerows, cattle, sheep, etc., all completely defined. In contrast was the special exhibition of modern art, where a sheet of black paper was entitled *Dark Study*. My sympathy went to those who can appreciate this form of bumbledom. An exposed Egyptian Mummy was a prize exhibit and the stuffed zoo contained a wide selection from the dormouse, moles, rats and wild cats up to a very impressive Irish wolfhound.

With the persistence of the wet weather, plans to visit Sligo out west were abandoned and on Sunday all the camp gear was again loaded and we set off for the frontier – rather a comic opera affair, where no one seemed unduly worried about who did what, except that you acquired a label to display in your windscreen, but a Morris Minor van going south was causing a little concern for the driver was required to alight and open the back of the van, whence out jumped a brown bear – on a chain!

On through Drogheda and into Dublin, where we rode all around one camp site and decided we did not like it so pressed on south out of the city to Shankhill which proved a very useful base for the next four days.

The weather in Dublin was far kinder in the lea of the Kennedy visit and this encouraged trips out to Wicklow, Arklow, the Japanese Gardens at Kildare, the seven churches of St Kevin at Glendalough and walks along the promenade at Bray. All too soon it was Thursday morning and everything was taken down, stowed away again and back we went to that frontier post, this time via Ballyboghill. Proceedings in this direction were a little less comic, as certain duty free items were available in the Free State, but if you had a clear conscience there was little delay.

We were back in Belfast in time for lunch and after a visit to the port office in the afternoon, returned to Ballynafeigh House for tea and dignified farewells to the owners who had gathered there to bid us adieu.

Once on the dockside, the curtain rose on a pantomime. The laden van was driven away to be loaded by crane deep down in one of the holds and the dock porters viewed myself and wheelchair with some concern.

'Cabin number sixty? That's second class, down four flights of stairs, dunno 'ow we're gunner getcha down there!'

'Wheelchairs are made to go downstairs, no trouble at all.'

'Can't take that thing downstairs, nothing to get hold of, have to use our chair', and off they go for a stroll round the dockyard. A little later a resounding rumble over the cobblestones heralds their return with the official dockyard chair, a monstrous brute of great vintage that should have been in the Transport Museum. It boasted a stud upholstered seat and full length stretcher handles all in heavy polished timber and the whole was mounted on four large cast iron wheels each of which must have weighed as much as the Dingwall wheelchair they so despised.

'If you want it that way, George, you can have it and the best of Irish . . .' So I climb aboard this leviathan sedan chair and off we went.

Passing the long queue of emigrants at the foot of the gangway, that always present dear old lady was heard to say, 'Makes yer thankful, don't it!'

Have her toes, George, that will calm her down. Up the gangway, along the deck and through the hatchway into the saloon, that was easy, but here comes the first flight of stairs with a rightabout turn landing half way down. I wonder how we'll get round there, but that's your worry, George. I'll grunt for you, if its any help. The breathing got deeper, the chair was on end, the ship suffered some damage and we were over that hazard, but there were three more to go. We negotiated the second landing and by the third, George appeared in a state of near collapse.

'You are heavy, sir' he gasped.

'So are those cast iron wheels, you silly boy. Mush, mush!'

Eventually we descended to the depths and there was

cabin sixty. They put me down outside the door with the prize remark,

'You won't go away, will you?'

The steward appeared with the keys, unlocked the cabin and I was in and it took just a few minutes to register that the temperature was rather high and that the diesel engine was right next door. Moral – never travel second class.

Landing at Heysham in the early hours of the morning, we decided on a long ride home, along the front at Blackpool, just as the 'bed and breakfasters' exited past the aspidistras. On to Liverpool just to sample the Mersey Tunnel and eventually to lunch in Denbigh, for our destination was Beddgelert, a Forestry Commission camp site in Snowdonia, where we spent the night. Saturday dawned bright and clear over the mountains of Wales to make a cheery end to a grand holiday trip, but by mid-day we were back again in the rain on one of the wettest days southern England had had for a long time.

We continued with camping holidays until 1964 when we loaded the van for what was to be our last encounter with the great outdoors and our first experience of Motorail. Leaving work at Victoria at 5.30 pm I drove the trike home to Wembley, had a quick wash and a bite, before we loaded the A35 van with our gear and drove off to Kings Cross and the Motorail terminal in the cattle dock off the Caledonian Road.

The cars travelled in covered vans with end doors forming a sort of tunnel, the second and third cars in each van being lowered between the bogies to load two more above and we took an ambulance chair as the only means of my being loaded into and wheeled along the corridor of the sleeping car from whence it was just possible to transfer the body through the compartment door and on to the bottom bunk. We pulled out of Caledonian Road at 9.15 pm and rattled onward through the night, pausing in York, Newcastle and Waverley, out over the Forth Bridge and into Perth at 6 am where on the adjacent track stood the royal train with a resplendent 'Duchess' class Pacific at the head. A very frustrating incident as I was quite unable to get up and out of the sleeper before the royal train pulled away.

The large Victorian toilets on Perth station were still in working order and clean, and their very spaciousness with

massive doors and solid wooden seats proved invaluable
before we retired to the station buffet for an excellent
breakfast of cereal, bacon, eggs, etc. It was then that we
trailed up the long slope to the road outside, over the bridge
and round to the car unloading bays where the A35 was
waiting ready for the road.

We climbed aboard, loaded the wheelchair and the
ambulance chair in the back and set off on the A9 out of town
towards Dunkeld, Pitlochry, Blair Atholl and eventually
Kingussie, Newtownmore and Aviemore where we turned
eastward up Glen More to the Forestry Commission camp site
on the shores of Loch Morlich. We set up the tent and got the
paraffin stove going by lunchtime – and I did not leave
Victoria until nineteen hours before – the cost of Motorail
sleeper return from London to Perth was then £28 for the van
and two persons.

It was a beautiful week there in the glen and the one
abiding memory of this large camp site was to be inside the
tent and hear a neighbouring camper arrive with a bucket of
water conveying a live trout, just out of the loch and offer a
tasty morsel to Enid. As she was a little uncertain of cooking
procedures for trout on a paraffin stove, I was sorry to hear
her say,

'My husband does not like trout!' despite the fact that he
had never had trout before.

At the end of the week we broke camp and drove out to
Kyle of Lochalsh to set the tent up in a quiet site two or three
miles before the port itself in this pleasant little village
opposite the Isle of Skye. Sunday was brilliant and we spent
the day high above the waters of Loch Carron where the
railway line runs along the shore on what really is the road to
the isles, that shows you the real beauty of those isles
particularly in the setting sun of a fine summer's day.

Climbing into the sleeping bags that night we were quite
unaware that the next three days would divert us from
camping for ever. By Monday morning it was raining hard,
so we made our way down to the water front and sat in the
van to avoid the weather. At lunch time we dashed into a
very convenient and clean looking restaurant that stood on
the edge of the railway line on one of the road bridges over
that line. A little light lunch strung out as long as possible and

then back to the van to shelter from the incessant rain. Tea was also taken in that same restaurant and prolonged for the same reason as was lunch, before we returned to the camp site which was by now well waterlogged. The damp atmosphere made even the sleeping bags none too warm, but we hoped for better things on Tuesday which in its turn was a repeat of Monday's escapades. On Tuesday night, with rain still hammering down, I elected to try sleeping in the sleeping bag in the back of the van, but this proved to be even colder than the tent.

Wednesday morning saw the rain continuing unabated, so we loaded the tent and all the gear in the back of the van – it was to be for the last time – and drove off towards Inverness and Perth in the vain hope that we might get on that night's Motorail, one day earlier than booked. The train loader in chief was fortunately sympathetic and managed to re-arrange his schedule by loading three 'little 'uns' where he had planned to place two 'big 'uns'. Never did we find out what he did with the 'big 'uns' but a sleeper compartment was made up and we were away from Scotland on the last of our nine camping holidays.

The main road from Kyle was under reconstruction and this served to fracture the exhaust on the van so it was providential that we arrived home on Thursday morning with time to have a new exhaust system fitted before setting out on Friday for Llanelli and the DDA Annual General Meeting on Saturday with return home on Sunday.

That AGM was attended by Lady Megan Lloyd-George and Jim Griffiths MP with whom we had our photographs taken for the local paper. Two schools were taken over for the weekend, one for the meeting and one for accommodation where civil defence beds were laid out in the classrooms and it was to one of these classrooms that I retired early on Friday night to settle down to sleep alone among the host of empty beds.

It was in the early hours of the morning that I was aware that the bed was gently rocking to and fro, that the light was on and a soft Welsh voice was apologising for waking me, but I would have to be moved. I climbed into the chair, the St John Ambulance man wheeled me out, while a nurse brought my clothes and the 'mechanical man'. At the door stood Ivor

Jones, who was the organiser of the weekend, tears stood in his eyes as he begged forgiveness for waking me and I was wheeled into another classroom. As the light went on, heads shot up in the beds around, but not a face did I know and their pained expressions in a Liverpudlian accent explained why. As I climbed into a clean bed, someone asked whence I had come and I replied 'Class II', which produced puzzled expressions all round before the next member was wheeled into the classroom. It was Johnny Johnson, who had got lost on the way to Llanelli and since one of his passengers was a lady, the only room they could vacate for her was Class II, which explained the situation.

Next morning Enid was up bright and early and went rushing into Class II to get me out of bed to be faced by Kathy and Julia sitting up in their beds and saying

'Good morning, Enid!'

Tea on Saturday was provided by the Town Council – chicken salad, strawberries and cream, etc – but before we started Jim Griffiths said a few words of welcome and gave a promise that 'We will sing to you before you go!' With tea finished Jim Griffiths called on a little bald headed man to lead the singing. He rose to his one foot and began to sing in a deep crisp base voice 'Land of my fathers' to which all Welshmen present immediately responded and the WVS, Civil Defence and Guides working in the kitchen all stopped work to stand in the serving hatchways and sing lustily and long as we had 'Men of Harlech', 'There'll be a welcome' and many more of the rousing songs of Wales, sung as only Welsh folk can. A truly memorable experience.

13

Moving

Since our marriage hard saving had continued and in 1958 we began viewing bungalows in the area, an exercise that eventually led us to a 1929 detached bungalow with garage and own drive near Sudbury and a mortgage was arranged on the purchase price of £3,300.

Chocolate paint and chair rails, embossed wallpaper and a selection of arctic glass, were all part of the deal and so we set about an extensive programme of DIY updating. The work had to be carefully organised into who could do what, but with the aid of a bench I erected in the corner of the big back room, a great deal was achieved between Enid and myself. The internal doors were removed, one by one, to be panelled on both sides with hardboard and fitted on the outside with long bar handles made from aluminium tee-bar, carefully patterned and polished with fine emery and duraglit wadding. This enabled me to close each door behind me with the added modification of roller catches instead of the old rim latches and knobs. At this time I was still on my feet with the aid of crutches and able to remove and refit the top hinge screws myself, doing the bottom ones by sitting on the floor.

The old French windows, double doors with small panes of glass, led out to the garden but not for me as the enormous threshold timber made a step some four inches high inside with a fifteen-inch drop outside which is one of the most awkward manoeuvres with crutches or a wheelchair. The solution was to sit on the floor and cut the centre portion from this great theshold strip, then to fill in the gap in the floor with floorboard, leaving a four inch gap under the doors. The next operation was the fitting of door extensions without removing the doors and this was achieved with face plates on both sides of the doors, which left just the eleven inch drop out of the doorway to the concrete path outside.

A rather forlorn glass verandah covered the back of the bungalow with rotting wooden glazing rails and small pieces of lapped glass in each panel. I set to with the production of a full set of aluminium tee bars made up from one inch by one eighth inch tee sections to screw to the eaves boarding and lay over to the existing timber outer rail of the verandah. My father was summoned to knock out the old glass, cut out the timber rails, clean and paint the gutter, the eaves and the top of the outer rail and then fix in place the new aluminium bars with new thirty-two ounce single panes of glass laid in putty. This was a major improvement but it still left the big drop outside to which the answer appeared to be a false floor and so we set to with a few old bricks and a bag of cement to build a line of brick piers on to which we laid timber joists and floorboards, to give a straight run out of the doorway for the wheelchair. The wooden posts of the verandah rail were then panelled in with hardboard inside and boilproof ply outside and from there I made up window framing to fill in the upper part of the panelling, giving glazing that leaned slightly outwards at the top.

I then set about making a pair of glazed timber doors to the construction method employed for steel doors at Art Metal and of course these were hung on substantial hinges with bolts, handles and a latch of the same ilk. The finished job gave me sheltered lounge space in my new garden and the next step had to be a timber platform outside the doors and a similar timber ramp down to the garden.

Of all the messy jobs we undertook, nothing was more unpleasant than the re-coating of the pebble dashed outer walls of the bungalow. We bought a small tin of Snowcrete, the whiter than white shade and conducted a few experiments on the back wall under the verandah using the recommended mixture applied with an old whitewash brush that bore the plain initials 'EAE' the one time property of Ernie Evans. The experiment on this scale seemed simple enough so we bought a large drum of white Snowcrete and started in the side alley obscured from the street by a high gate. Standing on a step ladder, Enid was able to cover the top half of the walls with the brush while I sat in the wheelchair below holding the bucket full of Snowcrete aloft.

This all seemed to work quite well as the steps were not the platform type and so could not support a full bucket, but after daubing away on a couple of yards of wall, it all became a bit like the old song of father papering the parlour, for the numerous drips, not to mention the occasional slosh that failed to get as far as the wall, all descended on me. By the time we had done the top half of the walls on all four sides of the bungalow, I had a collection of old clothing that stood stiffly to attention in a rock hard coating of white Snowcrete and a pair of boots that boot polish could not retrieve. It was also sad to note that the wheelchair, an MTP-8B, that was intended by its owner to be in a bronze enamel finish, was heavily splattered with Snowcrete that proved impossible to clean off even by scraping.

Never again did we ever attempt to brighten the outside walls of number 100 Charterhouse Avenue.

14

Journalism

My writings in the Minutes book in 1949 were less than as serious as Chairman Garry would have liked and it was said by a certain wit that the minutes were more entertaining than the newsletter and the obvious answer came to Garry, whence the exchange of jobs between minutes writing and compiling the newsletter were made.

It seemed to me that the newsletter needed a name and despite appeals for ideas, only Garry produced a single thought on the matter and so *Mrs Frequently* was launched and became a collated and stapled magazine. The title was a play on the spark plug problems we all had in those days and the content was a detailed report of each of our exciting and eventful trips to all points of the compass, plus our future ambitious programme. From the first issue in 1950 I drew strange cover designs for each succeeding issue and the first was a spark plug – the big 18 mm job – with the points splayed out as legs and an Ascot hat on the top – indeed 'Mrs Frequently' herself.

This design was drawn out on a wax stencil with a scriber and the typing of the other stencils was done by Don, who then ran off all the sheets on a flat bed duplicator, an extremely arduous task, before we collated, stapled and enveloped for posting. My handwriting and Don's typing combined to produce a galaxy of spelling errors that one member found so galling that he counted them up and complained bitterly. Ah well, you can but try!

In due course we bought a hand rotary duplicator with two drums so that we could produce two colour magazines and some frightful issues appeared after I took on the whole job of duplicating and mailing as well.

Mrs Frequently plodded on through the years and late in 1962, I had a visit from Jim Laffey, when he brought an invitation from the National Chairman, Denny, to take on the editorship of the *Magic Carpet,* the quarterly national magazine of the ITA. New Year 1963 saw my first effort at the production of a full printed magazine with an eight inch by five inch layout that ran eventually to eighty pages to every issue. The work was very interesting, for not only was it required to collect and/or write the content, but to do the full paste-up as well.

My first effort must have made the printer in Brighton cringe for having seen the galley proofs for the first time, I immediately cut off all the identifying marks and galley numbers and built the pages to the nearest line on each sheet. The issue was accepted with good grace by most of the membership and I continued with the *Magic Carpet* – having bequeathed *Mrs Frequently* to Jim Laffey – for six years, when I felt that the strains of travel to Victoria, a full day's work all the week and the intriguing business of the *Magic Carpet* were a little too much. So I resigned as editor and passed the whole business over to Bob Parker who had been a regular and dependable contributor for years past.

During my early years with the *Magic Carpet,* Denny, who always seemed to be my most loyal supporter, decided it was time for him to give up as National Chairman to make way for someone else, who fortunately was a friend of mine from Rochdale, Fred Needham. The other big change in the Association at that time was the demise of our first paid Secretary and the appointment of a new man in that position. He came from one of the local groups with ideas which I found incompatible with the past happy running of the ITA.

Our office was a freehold pre-fab bungalow in a rather rough area of Hackney with a couple of local girls working there. This modest but economic establishment was far below the dignity of the new man who immediately set about organising a management meeting in the bungalow and regrettably they fell for the line of inadequacy of the pre-fab and agreed to let him look for something more in keeping with his position as 'General' Secretary.

The result was the catastrophe of Blue Star House, where a

suite of offices on an upper floor was rented at the high price charged for such prestigious accommodation. Not only this, but it meant parting with Brenda, the East End girl who really made everything tick in the Hackney office.

Meanwhile I was writing reports of AGMs for the *Magic Carpet* and a few anecdotes would not come amiss.

In chapter seven are a few details of that first AGM in the schoolroom in Edgware and since that time such meetings have been held every year as required by law. Over those years the venue has changed constantly and the little episodes of humour that have arisen at those meetings are worthy of note.

On a beautiful Saturday afternoon, we were gathered in the Kodak Hall at Wealdstone to hear the National Chairman present his report for the year which included statistics of the rate of membership of the Association, in an effort to boost confidence that we were indeed growing and not fading away. When the Chairman invited questions from the floor, he was assailed by an elderly gentleman sitting on the window sill at the back of the hall. Mr Nichols was a member of the Surrey group and he proceeded to quote figures from the Chairman's reports of previous years, adding and subtracting as he went, to prove to his own satisfaction that these figures did not balance out. The floor were quite unable to assimilate the figures at the speed with which their delivery came and so they sat back in awe as Mr Nichols came to his punch line and he roared out 'What have you done with those 365 members, Mr Chairman?'

The platform fell silent as the hall and no answer came, as this was the age of the ready reckoner and not that of the calculator.

At Keele University, the meeting turned to the maintenance of our holiday hotel, Ashwellthorpe Hall as a viable proposition and from sundry speakers it seemed clear that this meeting might well vote to sell our one treasured asset in the heart of the Norfolk countryside, until an elderly member from West London came to address the meeting. He was hardly an elegant figure slumped in a wheelchair and he had a reputation for telling rather unbelievable stories and on the side of his trike, an 'Acedes', he had a tiny sign board which said 'The Flying Pig'.

Unknown as an orator, despite his stories, Mick Dicker launched into a major assault on the opposition to save the Ashwellthorpe Hall that he so obviously loved and enjoyed. So profound were his words that the whole meeting swung behind him and Ashwellthorpe lived to serve us many another day.

A similar situation arose when the meeting was held at RAF Locking, near Weston-super-Mare. A tirade from a member produced a vote to defeat the Treasurer's Report, which technically is a vote of no confidence in the auditor and this threw the platform into disarray before they adjourned the meeting for lunch and to give a little time to ponder the procedural rules.

Alexandra Palace was a regular venue for AGMs for many years and it was here that the attendant endeavoured to restrain a lady from bringing a Scots terrier into the hall, to which the lady replied indignantly

'But little Pongo has not missed an AGM yet!'

One of the failings of all DDA meetings was the wayward nature of the amplification equipment and the roving microphone that allowed delegates to address the gathering from the floor of the hall and Alexandra Palace was no exception, when the provider of the equipment sat in the hall with his control panel complete with knobs and buttons. It just happened to be the Queen's official birthday when the Trooping the Colour ceremony was taking place on Horse Guards Parade and as our Chairman was holding forth at our meeting, his voice trailed away and the Guards' Band was heard to be giving a spirited rendering of Colonel Bogey direct from Whitehall SW1! No explanation or apology was forthcoming from the operator of the equipment and we were left to assume that it was his sense of humour that led him to twiddle those knobs at that moment.

Of all the AGM stories, the best was yet another day at Alexandra Palace when the meeting was hammering one of its real chestnuts with further demands for the Minister to make numerous improvements to the trike. The topic was instability in cross winds on exposed sections of the highway and a lot of people had a lot to say about this until a Middlesex group delegate came to speak. This elderly lady, an inveterate trike driver, struggled to her feet in the centre of the hall and uttered those few words for which Dorothy will always be remembered.

'Mr Chairman,' she said, 'of course, we are all affected by the wind!'

The discussion sank deep into merriment and the Chairman had some difficulty in restoring order, but this episode must surely rank as the gem of our Annual General Meetings.

In 1954 the Annual General Meeting considered a resolution submitted by Middlesex group and dreamed up by Garry Nightingale, asking that the Association give support to the idea of acquiring 'holiday accommodation for disabled people'. The theory being that you can raise money for bricks and mortar far more easily than you can for administration.

The meeting accepted this idea with enthusiasm as the only available accessible accommodation for holidays then existing was the Infantile Paralysis Fellowship Lantern Hotel in Worthing which many of us had frequented in recent years. The inevitable sub-committee was commissioned and detailed plans laid before the survey of estate agents' offerings began. Chalets, bungalows, caravans and so on were considered and inspected, and duly rejected until that momentous day in 1957 when we were told of our purchase or rather, our mortgage that was to be set against our fundraising programme. In the quiet remote countryside of Norfolk, that area of East Anglia that can be so bleak and chilly, we were now the proud owners of a twenty three acre estate that contained a manor house with moat surrounding it, with its present occupant about to retire to South Africa on the proceeds.

The sum committed was £4,500 to include the gardener and a mangy old cat – together with the problems of the property itself. On hearing the news that we were a property owning organisation, everyone who could make it planned a day trip to Norfolk to see the site and some seemed to think they would find a fully functional hotel awaiting them without a second thought to the purchase price. Many were bitterly disappointed as they toured the dirty, decrepit and rotting interior of Ashwellthorpe Hall, others were full of the possibilities that it offered for the future, but it would obviously be hard work to bring the whole or even part of the building round to a wholesome standard of welcome to anyone.

Ashwellthorpe was a small village eight miles south of Norwich in the fork between the main London and Ipswich roads and the Hall, an ancient building dating from the days of Elizabeth I and substantially extended in Victorian times, has a long history of strange occupants, but none surely stranger than the DDA in 1957.

Weekend working parties of volunteers were gathered together to spend their time washing and scrubbing everything from the floors to the cornices, after removing a lot of the furniture to the garden and tearing down the heavy old drapes that graced the three front bay windows and other like places. As these drapes came down, so did the myriad of dead flies, bluebottles and wasps with plenty of spiders. The upholstered furniture was in the same state and the lot was consumed by a large bonfire in the grounds as soon as possible.

Straightforward cleaning was the order of the day, just to see if there was decoration underneath, but redecoration could not then be considered because of the limited time available to the volunteer force of mums, dads, wives, husbands, brothers, sisters and so on, who set out for Ashwellthorpe on so many weekends during 1958. Middlesex group were in the thick of this work but the efforts made by so many brave souls in those days go unrecorded or remembered and more is the pity! DIY holidays were instituted with sundry items of furniture purloined, bring your own bed linen and food, all at a modest charge per night – it was rather like weather protected camping!

By 1962 we had an offer to provide managerial and cooking services for the cost of the keep of the couple involved. Arthur Kingett came to retire from his employment and he and his wife Ella made this generous gesture 'for a couple of seasons' and so it was that they moved in the Hall in late 1962 and began preparing to accept paying guests and organise the ceremonial opening on 11 May 1963.

An enormous crowd of folk arrived for the opening day with all the locals plus a dozen coachloads from all around the DDA. The ballast of the terrace became a quagmire in the rain, the mud was tramped through the house by all those either desirous of inspecting the Hall or finding a usable toilet. The actor, Rupert Davis of Maigret fame, arrived late in a large American car and performed the opening ceremony by striking a match on the Gothic front door and lighting his pipe as the door opened. We were in business with basic limited staff and limited provision for guests!

Over the years there have been trials and tribulations but, we remain, at the time of writing, very much in business and filling a valuable spot in the holiday market for all disabled people, despite a considerable financial loss on the operation, due in large part to the maintenance of an ancient building, that could now well market at half a million pounds for the remaining eighteen acres and the interior improvements and extensions that we worked so hard to achieve.

After those six years and twenty four issues of the *Magic Carpet*, I retired and sat back for a rest, but returned for a second spell in 1978, during which time I managed to churn out 'A Brief Pictorial History of the Invalid Tricycle' as a feature in Spring 1985.

My second retirement was shortlived and twice more I went back to maintain continuity of publication of our quarterly national journal. During this time I was urged to produce a questionnaire on electric wheelchairs and battery powered scooters, to be followed by a detailed analysis of the 200 replies. The computer addicts said it would be simple – 'you just count the ticks!' was the advice, but in reality, every reply was covered in copious notes that were all eventually reviewed in 'The Electrifying Experience' in the Summer 1987 issue.

With promised final retirement at the end of 1987, I had completed fifty six issues of the *Magic Carpet*.

15

Decline

With less than competent management of Art Metal, the business began to slide and in February of 1972, the General Manager fell dead from his office chair and before that chair was as cold as its occupant, a new face from the accounts office stepped in and sat down. The new man's opposition to the partitioning business was obvious from the start and rumours of takeover of the company were being heard on all sides.

Takeover day was 1 August, when another firm bought the Art Metal business and immediately closed the Victoria factory. In the prior months, equipment was sold off and as the large presses, shears and brakes disappeared, the machine shop became a garage for employees' cars and it was then that I was persuaded by a junior in the office to take my car, by then a Bedford Beagle, up to Victoria to move two surplus desk pedestals that he had acquired.

The Beagle stood in the line of cars in the 'garage' and at lunch time in the canteen, a gentleman sidled up to me and whispered

'Have you seen your car?'

He winked and walked away. I had given the junior the car keys and told him to load the pedestals, two for himself and two for me. Descending in the lift at 5.30 pm, the cars came into view and the new General Manager and his stooge were walking along the line inspecting the vehicles. The Bedford had never been seen there before and my parking permit with my name on it was displayed in the windscreen and as she came into view, it was all too obvious that a very full load was on board. No less than seven pedestals and a selection of

132

other items of interest were on board and there were some problems in loading the wheelchair in the back, but it all worked out and we stopped at Shepherds Bush to offload all but two of the pedestals and the wheelchair.

The last trip to Victoria at the end of July was uneventful and the staff were spread over other sites. George, my most recent colleague, went to Queen Victoria Street, while the majority of the drawing office moved into a new office built with partitioning at the bottom end of the Wembley factory and I had a board and a desk adjacent to the cubicle occupied by Ron Lessells, the Chief Engineer.

The process of dissecting the firm was in hand and one by one different lines of production were being dropped from the range and by 1975 the drawing office was closed and the staff dispersed. Ron Lessells went to Southall with two others and I was moved, drawing board and all, up to the general office, that last saw a lick of paint just after the war. With Ron in Southall, George now in Bruton Street W1 and myself at Wembley, the problems of running a practical partitioning business mounted considerably, but we pressed on with Ron taking less part in the business which was left largely to George and myself, who liaised by telephone on customer problems.

George continued with site surveys and letter writing, we both did quotations and I did layout drawings, summaries and detailing for the shop, progress chasing and orders to the two sub-contractors. Other management provided little support or encouragement to us but we struggled on until the week of the Queen's Jubilee for which we were allowed the week off and on return, I was quite shocked to find that Ron had collapsed and died, so ending my close association with him totalling almost twenty five years. Management made no mention to me of Ron's death, such was their general apathy and when the day of the funeral came, I absented myself without a word to a soul and made my way to Ruislip Crematorium, where I met George and some other members of the staff for the brief service in the chapel at Breakspeare Road.

Returning to the factory again, no word was uttered as to where I had been for the last couple of hours or so and George and I were left to plod on with the business alone –

even to chasing the bad debts. Things were sinking quite
rapidly by now and a few months later, a fourteen inch block
wall was built across the factory and half of the floor area let
out to an Italian bakery, with the catchy name of Panificio
Italiano.

In July 1979 George collapsed in the street shortly after
leaving home in Byfleet for work one morning. He was taken
home, the doctor called and hospital examinations followed,
which led to a long and tedious series of tests and pill courses
that seemed to achieve little to reduce his blood pressure and
palpitations. The company were unsympathetic, they honoured his pay cheque for July and at the end of August sent
him a token payment. He remained quite unable to work and
as Christmas approached a food parcel from the office in
Bruton Street was delivered to be followed by a letter from
the company telling him that they intended to terminate his
employment and they would make him an honorary payment of £250 from which they would deduct their August
payment.

So much did the company care for a too diligent employee
who produced and submitted quotations to customers, who
did site surveys and customer interviews and was required to
visit any such customer who complained about the quality of
any installation when it was completed. This was often a
hazardous and unsavoury operation when the gentleman
concerned could well be poised for quite a showdown and
the company and George would have to meekly eat humble
pie.

So it was that at the end of September that year I was
engaged in another business meeting with the Managing
Director of the company, allegedly a millionaire. Driving a
succession of Rolls Royces, he always seemed to be unable to
grasp the realities of the factory floor and the dreadful mess
the whole place was in, while being totally obsessed with
statistics. His catch phrase could almost have been

'I must have the figures!' which he yelled as he came into
the office – it was not unlike Sandy Powell saying,

'Can you hear me, mother!' and his every decision was
based on the tables and charts and other statistics placed
before him by his minions, none of whom could muster any
bite at all.

After discussion of a job then in hand at Brooke Hospital, Woolwich, our boss relaxed slightly from his usual frigid manner, to talk of the future of partitioning in the company which really meant that as a production line it was finished. This led him on to tell me that he was proposing to make me redundant – a word I had long hoped to hear – and that I would be free to go at Christmas. The grapevine told me that I was expected to burst into tears and plead for my job, but nothing was further from my thoughts, as I could hardly wait to get out and away from such a torrid atmosphere as existed in the works. I departed at the festive season with a redundancy payment of six months' salary – that had not been increased for two years – and one day's holiday pay, after completing thirty six years and one week with the company.

In the weeks before my departure from Art Metal, an 'Auntie' like lady arrived in the office and announced that she was the DRO, a post in the Department of Employment intended to find employment for disabled people. We had a quiet chat in a private office and the lady listed my achievements and abilities and assured me that there should be no difficulty in finding me another position.

Her next question was, where did I think I might get a job, which dispelled any of my formed ideas that this lady was conversant with placing disabled people in employment – a job for which she was reasonably well paid and allegedly trained. I suggested Remploy in Cricklewood to which she responded enthusiastically and immediately telephoned Remploy Personnel Department and endeavoured to 'sell' me. At the conclusion of that call she said

'The moment I hear something, I will be in touch' and she was gone.

In January 1980, I began my own quest for a job by pursuing numerous advertisements, but no real joy was forthcoming by a combination of my fifty four years, my disability and the growing recession. Despite the 'Green Card' Act requiring employers to take three per cent of their payroll from the Disabled Persons' Register, my encounter at the Gas Board led me to a doctor's examination right there on the premises, whence I was told that my physical disability was no problem, but that my medical state would make me ineligible for their superannuation scheme, so that was that!

Sixteen weeks after Auntie's visit to the firm when she had promised to be in touch, I received a letter enquiring of my health and had I got myself a job yet? A certain animosity arose in my mind when I thought of the job she was supposed to be doing and my written response was terse.

Thirty-three job applications brought a few interviews for all kinds of work including the telephone enquiry department at the AA, where I was literally carried around the building, chair and all, shown everything that goes into the famous and intricate answering service of the AA, an immensely interesting experience and on the following day, I received a telephone call telling me that they did not think the building suitable for me, a fact that was all too obvious on my visit.

Eventually I filled in a Civil Service application form and was subjected to an intense medical examination at St Thomas' Hospital before becoming a Clerical Assistant or filing clerk in the great morass of the Civil Service. This could never be considered highly in job satisfaction terms but it is to be admitted that the company were all extremely amiable and helpful towards me, but it did confirm my opinion that a good Civil Servant will never say 'Yes' or 'No' in answer to any question without prior consultation with someone or something. My stay was brief and ended in March 1982 as related in another chapter.

My employment in the Civil Service was eventually ended on very generous terms and during my twelve months absence on sick leave, I was paid in full for the first six months and half pay for the second six months, which far surpassed the company's generosity in 1979. Five visits were paid to me by the PSA Welfare Department during that time, a Woolworth gift token for £10 was received at Christmas and after my retirement on health grounds, a repayment of my pension contributions plus a short term gratuity was sent to me and this made my Art Metal redundancy cheque look quite sick.

Thirty-six years as a draughtsman 'plus' contrasted strangely with my eighteen months as a filing clerk in terms of its reward. Little wonder there is no shortage of Civil Servants.

16

Medication

Everyone, particularly women, loves to talk about their ailments, real or imaginary, and discuss the learned statements about their condition as made by eminent men of the medical profession.

In my earlier days I went through the rigours of measles, mumps and scarlet fever and in each instance I was kept at home on the prescribed doses of the period. Scarlet fever came in 1935 and I enjoyed six whole weeks away from school, but the real disappointment came with the location of my bedroom in the front of the house with no view at all of the railway at the bottom of the garden, where the 'new works' programme of LT modernisation was then being plotted – a programme that would alter for ever, so many of the sights that had delighted me when we first arrived in Barnhill Road.

My health remained reasonable until the traumatic days of August 1938 and the aftermath already described. No additional major health problems arose until my daily journey to Victoria coincided with an over generous layer of pea soup fog, referred to by the popular press as 'smog', it being a direct by–product of a smoke laden atmosphere before the air pollution legislation intervened.

Exposure to this freezing morass of oblivion brought on a severe bout of bronchitis which came near to taking my breath away, but the late night attendance of Dr Arnold, our GP, produced some relief with an injection and the usual remedies took their time thereafter.

Over the years the odd nose bleed had been an inconvenience, but I gave no thought to the reason for these happenings until the Autumn of 1964, as I set to work scraping wallpaper off the bungalow walls. A severe bleed set in, brought about by the exertions and as it showed little sign of abating, a call was made to Dr Arnold which was eventually answered by a very unsympathetic stand-in. Lying on the bed without my structural steelwork, the doctor sniffed loudly, sat me up, grabbed my nose with finger and thumb in a vice-like grip and held firm for several minutes. When he let go, the accumulated blood flowed freely to make an awesome mess on me, the doctor and the bed. As this technique had obviously failed, he announced that he had a baby to deliver and he would return later.

When that later moment arrived it was midnight and my problems were still apparent so an ambulance was summoned and I was whisked away to Colindale Hospital where a blood pressure check was made with enquiries as to how much blood I had lost, and forthwith I was attached to the drip of a blood transfusion bottle. At a pint and a half, they decided to call it off, as somewhere along the line I had ceased to bleed and after a few days' rest in Colindale, I was deemed fit to return home and go back to work, without further check.

On a Friday afternoon in December the office at Victoria was ploughing through its work when another bleed started and dollops of cold water did nothing to ease the flow. With thoughts of my recent sojourn in hospital, the lads phoned for an ambulance into which I was loaded before the ambulance men held a serious debate on the merits of visual art portrayed by the female forms on duty at St George's and Westminster Hospitals. Westminster won and we were off to the accident unit in Horseferry Road where the immediate attentions of an over-zealous medical student were practised on me.

A large quantity of string-like material caked in what appeared to be kaolin poultice was inserted in my nose with a large pair of forceps and fed rather forcibly up past the large cavity of the nose until the gooey string appeared in my throat. The string was then packed tightly in the nose and all seemed well until the said student inspected my throat and declared he would have to start again – which he did! Then the Registrar appeared and after a preliminary investigation, he proceeded to take a blood pressure reading. His face fell into a very grave expression, he looked intently at me and said 'Have you got a life insurance?' I immediately thought the end was nigh, but no reassurance came except a promise of admission for further investigation, before I was whisked back to the ambulance for the short journey to Ebury Bridge. On the bridge, the trike stood waiting and I was helped into the driving seat, with the nose well plugged, a tickle in my throat and grim foreboding of what might happen next, as I trundled off into the darkness for the twelve mile journey home.

During the night the string substance worked its way down my throat and came out of my mouth with Enid cutting lumps of this string off as it appeared from my lips. Every movement caused a cough and more string emerged so that by morning a heap of cuttings lay on the bedside cupboard and any possibility of returning to Westminster Hospital for inspection was impossible. Dr Arnold was summoned, made sundry rude remarks about the packing of the nose and extracted the remaining string with no dire consequences.

Admission to Westminster soon followed and a three weeks' check list was worked through which produced the theory that hereditary tendencies had caused the problems that I could have expected at sixty – but I was only thirty-eight – and this was brought about by the poor circulation of long–standing polio. A hefty dose of pills seemed to work miracles and I returned to work after discharge on the day they buried Churchill, when London was at a standstill.

Life continued much as before as pills were consumed in large numbers, but on holiday in Derbyshire in the 1970s, a visit was made to Chatsworth House – well the grounds at least, as the house itself was not accessible – when the need for a toilet arose quite suddenly. It was decided to drive the six miles back to our base at Calver rather than risk problems struggling alone in the gents' at Chatsworth. We made it, but only just, and we decided it was the aftermath of some food partaken previously, but over the following year or so, more disaster struck due to the sheer physical effort required to move the body from the wheelchair through 180° to the toilet seat and struggling from there with clothing.

Many an embarrassing experience occurred and the

Westminster Registrar of that time was quite adamant that it was not the pills, until I was again admitted to the same bed in the same ward as before. A very uncomfortable eight days followed which proved nothing and soon afterwards a variation in the pill course cured all – instantly!

The basic theme behind the foregoing episode in my life is to illustrate that toilet facilities and their use pose great problems for many disabled people particularly when no immediate help is available in the loo itself. The Chronically Sick and Disabled Persons Act by Alf Morris MP, made access one of its main planks and the provision of public toilets for wheelchair users with sufficient interior space to turn a wheelchair, materialised as a major step forward in freedom of movement, but only in the unisex toilets of this kind could help be provided by another person.

All went well for a while until my last days at Art Metal when I developed bronchitis and was admitted to Northwick Park Hospital for a shot or two of oxygen followed by regular doses of a nebuliser, where a mask on an air line was applied and a small container filled with a gin-like substance was fitted to the bottom to provide aroma to the inhalant. Ignoring my respiratory problems, the doctor declared that I was overweight and moments later a dietician arrived to be followed by a starvation course, where the basic ingredient seemed to be large helpings of unsweetened tinned rhubarb, an insipid and overwhelming intake!

I returned to Northwick Park just twelve weeks later with a repeat dose of bronchitis by which time I had lost ten kilos, just over a stone and a half, and I really was so very much better for it.

All went well for a while and I plodded on with my duties as a Civil Servant, although much of what I was required to do was rather exhausting to say the least. In March 1982, I was driving the trike to work when the sight in my right eye failed completely – it was a very frightening experience! I turned the trike round and made slowly for home, driving on my left eye and after about a quarter of an hour, thankfully the sight in my right eye began to return and on reaching home I was alright, but very shaken, so I proceeded to see my GP who sent me to Westminster Hospital for a full works check.

The blood pressure had risen, probably by fright and the dose of hydrallazine was raised to 300 mg per day before I was despatched to Moorfields to be further viewed and yet another range of pills prescribed, before I returned home to make another visit to my GP.

Thoughts of retirement had been in my mind more recently, but I was anxious to be very much 'up and about' during that retirement, even so, it was a great surprise to find that my GP was writing out a medical certificate for six months and saying 'Go on, old man, retire and enjoy it!'

In contrast to the company, the civil service rushed their welfare department round to see me and to assure me that I would be paid in full for six months and half pay for another six months despite the fact that I had only been there for eighteen months all told! I brooded on my thirty six years at Art Metal and wondered where I had gone wrong.

Just before my holiday in June that year, a certain inconvenience in the chest appeared and I was admitted to a mixed ward in Westminster Hospital – quite an experience – where it was suggested that I had suffered a slight heart attack, but a reassessment of the pills stopped the bladder stimulant that drained me off and in five days I almost expired from lack of breath. Oxygen was applied and a draining substance injected that produced three litres of water in four hours! After that I felt better and the water pills were restored to the diet, but on being chest X-rayed, I was allowed to fall backwards in my chair and a severe crack on the head resulted – so they X–rayed my head as well!

The stay lasted three weeks and left me, for the first time, a little disillusioned with Westminster Hospital and I was tempted to consider if it was all part of the current campaign to dismantle the NHS that had done so much for me in the preceding thirty-four years.

The other item that the medical men were looking at was described as a 'pulsating mass' in my stomach and this was viewed, examined, measured and ultra-sounded, to come to the conclusion that the main artery was dilated, to which they all gaily said 'that's alright, we can put a piece of plastic pipe in there!'

My holiday in Wensleydale had gone overboard and so had one or two other interesting invitations that my retirement would have allowed me to accept, but the thought of that plastic pipe weighed heavily upon me. On a return visit to the hospital in August, I was further disillusioned by the registrar who told me that if the aneurism was to burst, that would be that. Anyway the operation was very, very serious and I might well die and even then my chest would not stand the anaesthetic! There seemed to be no way out.

We went home totally demoralised by the bland remarks and attitude of this man and took our troubles straight round to my GP. This produced a letter directly to the Consultant, followed by an appointment to view the body, where the aneurism was now clearly visible. The interview calmed the situation to a remarkable degree as this mature little man with Consultant status tried to explain the symptoms and the problems to me, despite the considerable handicap of a speech impediment that must have proved very difficult when talking to a gathering of young medical students.

'Go home now, rest up and come back and see me in twelve weeks' time', he said in hesitating tones. 'Meanwhile, we'll run a few tests and let the surgeon see you and I will give you a positive decision on whether we operate, when I see you again.'

The twelve weeks passed happily by, under growing apprehension of my next interview and on 7 December, that little man with the stutter said,

'I think it's time to start work', and I was admitted soon afterwards.

Two days later, I was whisked away to the scene of the action where the grapefruit sized bulge on my belly would be split open to have a length of plastic pipe inserted into the main artery as a sort of sleeve to bridge the offending and threatening bulge in the aorta. It was a four hour job where I was later told by an enthusiastic eye witness that everything was taken out, rearranged and put back before I arrived in the intensive care unit fitted up with plumbing to every orifice and to be kept in total sedation for another five days.

During this time, I dreamed seemingly endlessly and always it was a traffic scene that always involved the trike and in one of these fantasies I was approaching one of the big iron bridges that span the Great Western outside Paddington station, when a trike, a model 57 Acedes, zoomed in from the right hand side of the road, overtook a line of traffic on the nearside and shot out into that line when a space opened up. These were horrendous days for me and it is a strange fact that I never again expected to drive my beloved trike. A chapter of life was over – or so I thought.

At long last, I opened my eyes for real and there stood a nurse. 'I've seen you before' I said and I was back in the real world and the operation was considered a success. But joy was not for long, as three days later I found myself fighting for breath in a terrifying episode before I passed out completely. It was Christmas Eve and while I was rushed back to the Intensive Care Unit, an urgent call was sent out to Enid to attend and when I did eventually surface again, I found a ventilator rammed down my throat, holding my mouth open wide which was distinctly uncomfortable, to say the least, but I was still in the land of the living if only just.

ICU was all subdued lighting and the adequate staff seemed to spend most of their time re–arranging and renewing the miles of plastic plumbing attached to every patient. While this went on, we were honoured by a visit from Basil Hume, the Archbishop of the nearby Westminster Cathedral, in full stand down regalia.

On 8 January, just twenty five days after admission, I was sent home and never was home more wonderful.

17

IYDP

When 1981 was declared to be the International Year of Disabled People, we all wondered what it would bring and for myself it proved very interesting indeed.

Working on paste-up of the *Magic Carpet* on Good Friday, I was troubled with inconvenience in my chest and this remained with me on Easter Saturday morning, so I sought an appointment with my GP who after superficial examination, phoned Westminster Hospital to seek their advice and forthwith, I was en route for Horseferry Road.

In the Casualty Department I met the duty Registrar who ran an ECG on me after examination and declared that the readings were very different to the last chart in my file.

'Go home, have a quiet weekend and I will see you again on Tuesday,' he said, so we retreated to the foyer to sup a cup of tea, when an arm fell on my shoulder and the Irish lilt of the Registrar said, 'I've been thinking, perhaps you had better stay for a few days, in case . . . '

In case of what? I thought, but not for long, as I was wheeled up to Edgar Horne Ward on the third floor and straight into bed – the same bed in the same ward that I had occupied twice before.

Having been attached to a monitor, a sort of VDU screen that gave constant zig-zags of the heartbeat, I was definitely there for the Easter weekend. By Monday I was permitted to visit the toilet, so I unplugged myself and departed, but was rather alarmed to note on my return that the screen on the locker was still producing a trace. I climbed back into bed and plugged in again, which made just no difference to the screen; it went on with its zig-zags just as before. On the next appearance of the doctor, I mentioned the incident in the hope of an explanation, but he was quite unabashed and said, 'Oh, yes, we are watching the KGB on there!'

All was considered reasonably well after my weekend stay and I returned home bewailing my lost Easter weekend, but by Spring Bank Holiday recompense was at hand. The Swedish car company, SAAB, advertised a revolving seat in their car as an aid to a disabled person and I wrote for details and a photograph for use in the *Magic Carpet*. Their reply offered me a few days' trial of the car, which sounded very interesting indeed, so I hastened to phone SAAB in Marlow where the response was an enthusiastic, 'When would you like it?'

I sat back and gasped for a moment before I suggested Spring Bank hoiliday weekend, to which the immediate answer was,

'We'll deliver on Friday and collect on Tuesday. How's that!'

I could not believe my luck until it arrived; a maroon SAAB 99 with automatic gearbox, power steering, cruise control, quadraphonic radio, electric windows, revolving driving seat and SAAB hand control gear. The fact that the car was left hand drive with Swedish registration was a complication, but the SAAB representative was quite placid.

'Sign here,' he said in an unconcerned manner without asking to see my driving licence or mentioning insurance.

I managed to get in a brief buzz round the block before he departed, whence he said,

'If you are not here when I collect on Tuesday, just shove the ignition key up the exhaust pipe, that will be alright!' and he was off.

I viewed the handbook and the literature and ascertained that this car would sell at upwards of £8,000 so we decided against placing the key in the exhaust pipe!

We got five hundred miles in that weekend and very enjoyable it was too, indeed a thought to be weighed against my Easter weekend.

At this time another invitation arrived to lunch at Ragley Hall with Lord Hertford for the launch of the Elswick Envoy, a little wheelaboard car that could be driven sitting in a wheelchair. It was just a hundred miles to Ragley Hall, where

I was man-handled up the ornate stairway and into the state room with log fire burning brightly in the enormous fireplace and on the carpet, a sheet of polythene to protect it from any drips from the car that stood in the centre of the room. The whole business looked like a terrible fire hazard to me and as the car had been dragged up the flight of steps from the terrace outside, it was not going to be a quick job to get it out again in the event of problems.

However, I cast these thoughts from my mind and set out to cross question the Managing Director of the car manufacturers on the points I hoped to raise in my report for the *Magic Carpet*. Having achieved my objective, the Managing Director turned on me to tell me that Lord Hertford would be saying a few words of welcome to the journalists present then he, as Managing Director, would tell the tale of company aspirations for the Envoy and he wanted someone to respond and would I do just that?

Oh dear, little time to think, certainly no time to write a script and his Lordship held the floor, followed by the Managing Director and I was on! I tried hard to sound confident of the success of the Envoy despite my doubts with a £7,000 price tag and then we all retired to lunch. By jingo, how the other half live! A sumptuous cold table was laid out for eager consumption and it caused me to wonder if journalists were journalists for the sake of the receptions and lunches to which they are invited. My friend from BSM was there adding to his waistline with relish and everything else on the table, all topped off with strawberries and cream!

Test drives were available after lunch and I elected to try the red sample car there for demonstration, but it had to be started on jump leads and the seat belt would not unwind, but apart from that it was really an excellent day and well worth the 200 mile round trip.

Later in the year I received another invitation of grand proportions to a Garden Party at Buckingham Palace in honour of IYDP. Alas the invite was only for myself without Enid, so I went by trike to meet the Queen. Approaching the Palace from the Royal Mews end, I was hailed by a WPC who told me that I should drive down the Mall and join the queue, despite the open gate in front of me. I trundled round Queen Victoria and into the Mall where a triple line of cars, cabs and coaches stood motionless facing the Palace. Almost at once I was hailed by a policeman who said,

'Go right down the Mall, right round Trafalgar Square and come back to join the end of the stationary queue.'

Having agreed, I trundled off and on reaching St James' Palace, a constable was controlling the traffic to let some vehicles out of St. James' and the opportunity loomed to do a swift U turn with the trike and I was in the queue!

The next policeman told me to stay in this line, which I did as we eased forward until I came to another police lady who had different ideas.

'You are in the wrong line' she said. 'Go down here, round the monument, back up the Mall, round Trafalgar Square and join the back of the queue.'

I felt that as the invitation was for THAT afternoon, I was in danger of missing out altogether, but I ambled forward and as I came abreast of the Monument with the winged figure above, it became obvious that the tail end of the previous contingent was just entering the gate and the solution was abundantly clear – tag on behind – which I did and was ushered to a parking place on the Palace forecourt.

As I slid the trike door open, a guardsman in stand-down uniform came up and offered to help and I was duly wheeled round to the garden entrance where an august figure in red-tailed coat and top hat took my ticket and we proceeded into the garden without security check of any kind in those days of much terrorist activity.

'Where to?' said my guardsman.

'To the wheelchair loo' I replied and away we went over the fine loose shingle to a discreet corner of the royal backyard where stood two plastic huts with sanitary interiors. I dismissed my guardsman, went in, performed and came out quite happy that I could push myself on the close mown lawn of Buck House, but the damp atmosphere was against me and I struggled mightily with the wheelchair on the damp soft grass until an elegant figure in frock coat and grey topper offered to push me. It transpired that he was an usher or he may have been an undercover man for MI5, but he pushed away towards the long pavilion that lines the left hand side of the garden and as we drew nearer he said,

'It looks like rain, you'd better go in here', and in there I was amid a selection of the customary garden party looking folk who in turn cast me some sympathetic glances.

The shower passed over and I ventured out of the hut and proceeded slowly along the front searching for a familiar face, which I eventually found. Several, in fact and greetings were exchanged before I came upon Wally Siggers sitting inside the pavilion who beckoned me in with a cheery welcome,

'Come in here, boy, I think it's going to rain.'

As we supped tea and fancy cakes from the long counter manned or womaned by 'Nippys', we watched as the guests gathered in long lines between the terrace outside the palace and the tea marquee down by the lake. Then the rain began to fall and by the stroke of 2 pm as the Royal party emerged on to the terrace the rain reached deluge proportions and brollies went up as a quick growing forest.

Wally and I watched the stately progress of the host party umbrellas as it did its dutiful walkabout between the two long regimented lines of guests with the odd bod here and there wandering about in a drenched daze around the lawns. Among this array of wanderers was a handsome lad in a wheelchair, who was dressed in full morning suit, soaked to the skin and pushing himself slowly across the sodden soft grass towards shelter in the pavilion. Obviously his great day was in ruins.

As we sat in the pavilion with the rain dripping into our cups of tea standing on the rail, the other braver souls were there hob-nobbing with the royal party that consisted of the Queen, Prince Philip, Princess Anne, Princess Alexandra, Angus Ogilvie, Prince Charles and Lady Diana, just one week before THAT wedding. There were many kind thoughts for Lady Di as she was seen to remove her glove for a blind guest to finger her engagement ring – still in the rain. A few favoured guests took tea with the Queen in the marquee while the long line outside waited for the rain to ease off, which it eventually did and I ventured out of the pavilion to be seized by an enthusiastic police cadet, who propelled me straight away to the front rank of the crowds still lining the 'walk back' route to the terrace.

Shortly afterwards, the official tea in the marquee was over and the host party set out on their return walkabout back to their homestead. The Duke and Lady Di strolled along the far side, Princess Alexandra criss–crossed from side to side having a word here and there, while the Queen and Charles covered our side of the gathering and just after passing me, it was the Queen who retraced her steps to enquire about my DDA badge. I told her that Prince Philip was our Patron, that he had recently been to one of our events at Canterbury Cathedral – by helicopter – and that brought the response that 'he loves his helicopter!'

The Yeoman Warders lined up in front of us as the Royals mounted the steps to the terrace and the head Pikeman was heard to say in a tired tone

'Alright then, quick march' and they followed the host party up on to the terrace where a final wave was produced before they entered the palace and the day was almost over.

Late in the year came yet another invitation, this time to the Design Centre in the Haymarket, where an exhibition of selected aids for the disabled was on display. The selectors were chaired by the Duke of Gloucester and it was he who opened proceedings for the assembled press men.

As the only disabled person present, I was pleased to have a chat with the young Mr Gloucester amid the exhibits and these few words clearly showed the commonsense approach he had to life and its problems for anyone with a disability.

Early in the following year, Toyota came up with another invite, this time to their new range launch at Goodwood House and so we made our way to the famous circuit to sample the new delights. The demonstration cars were gathered in the centre of the circuit and journalists were hammering many of these cars around the track at great speed, while access to the centre was via a subway under the track.

After a lengthy pause beside the track, a Toyota marshall raced the wheelchair across the track between the passing cars and we were there to view the display.

'Just take which car you like' said the head of operations, so we selected an automatic Corolla, climbed in and with Enid driving, we headed for the road circuit to have a very pleasant ride all round Chichester and the Sussex countryside without a question being asked.

Back at Goodwood, we viewed the Corolla Estate and persuaded another visitor to give us a couple of very high speed laps of the race track in a hair-raising ride after which we retreated to Goodwood House for drinks and an excellent five course lunch, all to the accompaniment of a steel band that was shaking the building of this stately home.

Such are the delights of life for the eminent journalist who is constantly entertained in this manner in an effort to obtain coverage of this or that product in the said journalist's publication. What a pity the *Magic Carpet* is such a lowly magazine.

18

The Interest

That 'source of interest in later life' referred to in Chapter 1 was always the railway, stimulated by reading all those railway magazines loaned to me in the war years. Visits to most of the places of interest and nearly all the myriad of preservation centres set up in the 1960s and 1970s have been achieved.

Bridges like the Forth and the Tay and less spectacular structures like Connel Ferry and Loch Creban, the concrete viaduct on Glenfinnan, Culloden Moor, Grant Castle and many lesser Victorian achievements in Scotland have all been viewed and photographed. The Royal Border bridge at Berwick and Bellah Viaduct in the North of England to the Brunel monument at Saltash, the Royal Albert Bridge and in Wales, one of the most impressive, the old Crumlin Viaduct, up to the rather mundane Barmouth bridge over the Mordach Estuary, as well as the Menai Bridges.

Bluebell was one of the first preservation centres visited, encouraged by their acquisition of the 'Chesham Set' of Ashbury stock from the Metropolitan, vehicles that I rode in from Wembley Park in the early 1930s and whose appearance remained little changed in their new surroundings.

When the Transport Museum was first opened in the old tram shed at Clapham Common, we all four paid a visit and paid the statutory shilling admission fee which got us into a little office block of the depot where a few models and tickets were on display. Three of us were able to go upstairs to look around while I remained downstairs chatting to the attendant who expressed some concern that I was unable to see all that was on show at that time. He went to his superior to tell the sad tale, whence my father and I were permitted a preview of the large exhibits section that was not then ready for display to visitors.

It was an excellent show of all forms of public transport and particularly interesting as work was still in hand on some of the exhibits prior to their full public viewing.

On holidays, odd visits were made to Buckfastleigh and Kingswear in South Devon and the West Somerset railway at Minehead, the loco on the pedestal in Tavistock, David Shepherd's centre at Cranmore, Bulmer's at Hereford, Ashchurch and the Severn Valley at Bridgenorth. All were scrutinised in the limited manner open to me as I was unable to take many of the paths or climb the footbridges and subways, although the Didcot Railway Centre, home of the Great Western Railway Museum provided a lot of manpower for me to climb out of their subway on the day that 'Pendennis Castle' arrived on its farewell tour before its sale to Australia.

There were many visits to the Bucks Railway Centre at Quainton Road Station, particularly to see Metropolitan No 1 where restoration ran at a pace for some years and then sadly appeared to cease altogether leaving the frames and under-carriage restored and the boiler to rust in the yard. But eventually No 1 was brought back to steam and looked just as she did from that bedroom window at Barnhill Road in 1931.

A brief visit was made to Wakes Colne, more attention being paid to gardens and exhibits at Bressingham where the Alan Bloom collection is on show. Sheringham was another interesting, if somewhat dilapidated centre and the King's scrap sidings at Ashwellthorpe turned up a lot of odd sights whilst in operation. There were quick glances at Nene Valley at Peterborough on numerous journeys up and down the A1, visits to York Museum even in its original form as well as to the new National Railway Museum with its great display and its exquisite models. While in Yorkshire we tripped up to Goathland and over the moors to Pickering and ventured further west to Carnforth and even Ulverston for Lakeside and on to the Ravensglass and Eskdale Railway coming down the back of Hardknott Pass.

Our railway experience in Wales is documented in another chapter and subsequent visits have taken us on the

Festiniog Railway into the new terminal in Blaenau Festiniog.

Other train journeys were few, apart from the Motorail trips to Perth on five occasions, but while in Scotland we boarded the Mallaig train at Fort William with the aid of an enthusiastic railwayman who helped to lift me into the guard's van and then charged the chair, with some force, into the entrance to the corridor where we came to a violent halt. I raised myself on to the armrests and part folded the chair so that we could progress down the corridor, where I was just able to squirm round the doorway to settle my bottom on the seat inside. Sliding up to the window seat, the railwayman sat down opposite to me and pulled the chair in behind me, while Enid went to buy two return tickets to Mallaig.

It was at the time of the building of the papermill at Corpach and my companion gave vent to his local feelings about the unsavoury characters imported from Glasgow for the construction work, who he suspected would stay on to take work in the mill when it came into operation, despite the publicity generated to imply that the mill work would be for the local folk of Fort William and around. In the midst of this tirade, a gentleman in a bowler hat appeared in the doorway of the compartment, whereupon my railway friend leapt to his feet and proclaimed this to be a reserved compartment and the gentleman retreated with profound apologies.

My friend also departed when Enid returned with the tickets and soon afterwards we were underway, out of the old Fort William station on the waterfront and bearing sharp left to cross the swing bridge over the Caledonian Canal. It was a leisurely and very pleasant journey along the shore of Loch Linnhe past the paper mill at Corpach that was planned to bring so much traffic to the railway and we ambled on through the beautiful western highlands occasionally coming within sight of the road, but at other times out in blissful seclusion that failed entirely to disturb the wildlife, such as the stag that stood and watched the train go by just as he had done for all his life without fear that the trundling monster would do him harm in any way.

At Loch Sheil, the railway crosses Glen Finnan on a long curving concrete viaduct of many arches and I was so busy panning my camera to the grimy carriage window where I obtained an excellent picture of the viaduct of many arches and the train sweeping round before me, that I forgot altogether to admire Bonnie Prince Charlie stood high on his pedestal down by the lochside, commemorating the landing of his small band before his defeat at Culloden in 1745.

We alighted from the train in Mallaig to smell the fish, wonder at the number of seagulls, partake of tea and watch the process of detaching the Beaver Tail Observation Car that once graced the Silver Jubilee Express out of King's Cross revolve it on the turntable and couple it to the rear of the train for the return journey to Fort William. At this stage, I hastened to raise my camera again as a porter arrived with a broom and a bucket of water and proceeded to wash the windows of the observation car for the benefit of those passengers who had paid the supplementary fare for the delight of riding in this all vision carriage at the end of the train.

A most enjoyable trip and one that I was truly pleased to make while the opportunity was still with us to enjoy a view of Scotland that the political Philistines may one day deprive us of.

In 1980, we took a self-catering converted cowshed at Lentran, some six miles beyond Inverness. The conversion was very comfortable and spacious and formed an excellent base for surveying a large area of Scotland and it was from here that we booked on the Kyle train out of Inverness one morning after the said Philistines had disposed of the old Devon Belle Observation Car that once trundled the line and been tempted to hire an even older Caledonian Railway Tail Coach from a preservation society, that was only partly able to fulfil its purpose, as the demise of the turntable at Kyle of Lochalsh meant that observation car passengers could only observe the back of the engine on the return journey when the setting sun over the western islands as the train pulls out of Kyle and runs along the coast through Plockton, is the real sight to observe on this fascinating journey through the wilder parts of the Highlands.

19

I wish . . .

With more than half a century behind me, I can look back over the years and muse over the things I have not done that I so wish that I had.

There was not much of life in Achilles Road that I remember apart from the gaslight and the little padded and rather realistic horse on cast iron wheels I trailed up and down the garden, so that there is little else I could have wished for, but with the great adventure of arriving in Barnhill Road with a Co-operative removal van, life became so much more interesting.

The horse disappeared at this time, to be replaced by my wheelbarrow, a sturdy all-metal job to be raced up and down the long garden over the rough farmland it had so recently been, but I wish I had been a little older then, that I could have taken a more detailed interest in the railway before the days of London Transport, have noted the haulage of the Great Central expresses to Manchester when so many pre-grouping locomotives were still on the road and been able to absorb more of the world about the City end of Metroland as it was in 1931.

Ah well, small boys must wait, I suppose, and I could have few regrets about life at Fryent School, but August 1938 changed all that and two wasted years ensued in the grasp of the medics.

How I wish I could have remained in Great Ormond Street Hospital where I was cared for so admirably, where I might well have remained without that damning spinal deformity, where I was and could have continued to be in good physical shape – and I mean proper shape, rather than the awkward posture that developed, in the wake of neglect on those dreadful wards at Stanmore. It was this deformity that dictated the construction, with all its size and weight, of the mechanical man previously described which they said was necessary for me to even sit up and the discomfort of which I had to endure every day of my life from my fourteenth year.

The pathetic construction of this equipment was just plain stupid and it came about because it was built up on the bench and grew like 'Topsy' without a thought for any prior design work on paper even of the most elementary kind. How I wish I had had the wheelchair and the mobility that the National Health Service eventually gave me and that I could have got my tuition at Leatherhead under my hat and then gone into the surgical instrument business as it was then called, but since uprated with the pompous title 'Orthotics'. Not that I could have done anything spectacular in that business, but my later experience clearly showed the problems of getting a little design work over on the alleged experts in the workshops. They seemed strangely unable or unwilling to understand a detail drawing of the hip pivot and stop device that I eventually proved to be a vast improvement on their unchanging Heath Robinson ideas.

My rather bitter feeling on this subject was the essence of an editorial that I wrote for the *Magic Carpet* in Spring 1964 –

'Ladies' fashions change annually at the great command from the font of the business – Paris – but this is no more than a money-spinning gimmick that is of no real practical importance to anyone. Other fashions change too and the fashion that is of increasing concern to many of our members is the wheelchair.

'It is not so long ago that every patient discharged from hospital had, by the demand of the fashion of the day, to be "on his feet", even if the effort were enough to all but lay him back and even when he stood on his useless feet, he was quite unable to do anything for himself or anyone else. You may have been carried in, but you had to go out on your feet; it was a matter of pride to the medical profession – if you were wheeled out there was only one destination.

'The efforts made and the methods employed to attain the vertical were often quite gruesome. The weird array of steel scaffolding erected around some of the bodies weighed more than the bodies themselves and the design, if it was designed, was painful in every respect. Most of it appears to have just "happened", to have materialised as construction went on; extra straps, steel bracing, buckles, screws and rivets, padding, binding and all the rest – like father decorating the Christmas tree. But you had to be on your feet, however much it hurt!

'Many of our members know about this first Victorian step to mobility and there is no one voice in the land to browbeat the brains behind this ironmongery, into making any sensational advance in its design. These same brains produced those hideous black boots with furlong laces, because there is no one to dispute their claim that they know best – except you and you are the patient . . . '

My time at Leatherhead was never exploited to the extent I would have liked as I never pressed or asserted myself on the system, where I could well have completed my drawing office time and taken a turn in the gas welding shop to extend my knowledge and experience of engineering and probably my chance of employment in the great race for war production at that time.

There is little doubt that my lifetime at Art Metal could have been more constructively used had I been more pressing and my attempts to find alternative employ were never sufficiently serious or determined in their approach, for the same reason. A lack of confidence to proclaim my own abilities which amounts to an excess of personal modesty that may disappear with these writings.

My wanderings in the hand propelled Trilox were never very venturesome either and usually over the same ground. There were few friends to visit within pedalling distance and my grandparents at Twyford Abbey was a fairly regular Saturday afternoon stroll to gaze over the Iron Bridge at Neasden on the way home, to survey the railway yard and what little would be happening there on a weekend.

With the acquisition of the Argson, great new horizons loomed and my biggest regret is that I did not invest in a better camera at the same time but continued to struggle with the big Brownie Box that belonged to my mother and took snaps $2\frac{1}{2}$ inches by $4\frac{1}{4}$ inches dimensions. It did produce some quite historic photographs, but to me the effort of peering down into the tiny view finder as I held the camera close to my chest, was a considerable disadvantage in the scope of pictures I could acquire. That camera travelled countless miles in the large steel box that I fitted under the seat of the Argson, together with a glass jar for personal relief. The steel box was of Art Metal manufacture including a desk lock to secure the valuable contents therein.

In the summer of 1948, before the Middlesex group was launched, I regret that I did not drag myself away from familiar beaten tracks; Wimbledon was always via Askew Road and Hammersmith Broadway to Putney Bridge, whereas Wood Lane/Scrubs Lane would have brought me to Mitre Bridge with a grandstand view of the Great Western and a lineside spot on that climb northwards from Olympia on the West London line and there were many other such places of immense interest in 1948 that escaped my gaze, as I stuck to my own well known tracks before Middlesex group dragged me away in all directions.

My photographs of those early days with the group were taken so sparingly that much of our venturesome and quite hectic travels remained unrecorded on camera. In the light of later experience, my miserly attitude to buying film for the Brownie at that time is another great regret to me, as pictures tell so much more than words ever could of those exhilarating days of 1949.

The same careful approach took us on our first camping holiday in 1956 where I could have snapped away happily at the delights of the age, but alas, I did not and it was not until 1960 that my meagre knowledge of cameras took me to a Boots chemist in Burnt Oak where a patient assistant explained the intricacies of a Kodak Coloursnap camera which I purchased for just £10. A distance scale in feet was included which held no problems for me and the aperture was controlled by a scale of four small squares indicating bright sunshine, hazy sunshine, dull and buckets of rain. A colour slide film went into that camera and we set out for the DDA Annual General Meeting at Giffnock to try it out.

Over twenty years have passed since then and the Coloursnap remained my only photographic equipment and it has produced some very good pictures in that time, but never with the snap-happy approach that my economic mind forbade.

Another aspect of my frugal attitude was my loyalty to Art Metal, a company that at no time really justified that degree of support and in latter years literally scorned its employees' devotion. The day of my grandmother's funeral in 1945 would have been my last opportunity to see many of the older generation of Nailers in Reading but I went to work at Art Metal lest the tale of Gran's funeral was met with scepticism. Much the same thing happened when my other grandparents died and so it went on with my old fashioned belief that my job depended on my attendance, so rapidly becoming the enigma that I failed to appreciate.

Life at the Civil Service was much the same for when an invitation came to attend a DHSS meeting in Blackpool to finalise their official Code of Practice for Construction and Use of Hand Control Gear on Cars, I felt unable to risk three days leave to attend, whereas a little gall on my part would probably have got official blessing for three days absence.

Like so many folk, I look back and wish that I had interrogated my relations for their memories and knowledge of past family history. Those stories of John Nailer's horse coming home without him to the cottage at Bucklebury where he lived. He was found in Bradfield Woods either robbed or drunk, depending on which story you chose to believe. How grandfather Fred walked to work from West Hampstead to St John's Wood followed all the way by Gran who was unable to catch up with his long legged stride to give him his vital sandwiches. When those sandwiches did reach his hand, grandfather Fred is reputed to have said,

'A good soldier never looks behind', whence Gran retraced her steps for home.

Another story of which I would have liked to know more is about one of the thirteen children of John and Mary Anne, who became known in Bucklebury as the 'Donkey King' for the collection or bevvy or whatever it is, of these big-eared creatures that he kept, for I know not why. And there was uncle George who had both legs amputated due to the effects of diabetes. When did this happen? Where was it done, and with how much butchery in those far off days?

I have made up my vast collection of old family photographs, for which I have to thank my father, into a family history album, as far as my limited knowledge of the distant past and my own memories of the 1920s and 1930s onwards will allow, but how I would like to fill in the gaps in pictures and information. One particular gem that seems to have disappeared at the ungracious hands of a maiden aunt, is the photograph that adorned the walls of their home in Twyford Abbey. An official posed photograph of grandfather David Harper 'up', as the expression of those days was, in the driving seat of his two horse bus in 1907, with the London Road Car Company.

Ah well, how I wish . . . '

20

The Morbid Side

During the years of the war there were regular letters from Aunt Lil telling of the fortunes of the Nailer family and every letter seemed to convey the tale of the demise of this or that aunt, uncle, cousin or 'in–law', but the full facts of death did not really reach me until 1945, just after the war ended, when my grandmother died.

She had lived with us for all my life, as my grandfather – Fred I – had died of a heart attack in 1907 while working on the St John's Wood power station and she was buried in his grave in Reading cemetery. The carriage at the funeral was to carry my mother and father only, but before the funeral left Wembley Park, Ernie Evans appeared on the scene to share that carriage, an act that was so typical of the thought he could always be depended upon to provide in time of need.

My father was, of course, executor of Gran's funeral and affairs and the following year his cousin, George Coates, died in Reading and in 1947 George's mother died and both these funerals and the subsequent tidying up fell to my father to carry out. This led my Aunt Ethel to make the unkind comment that 'Sid should put up his brass plate!'

My father had to clear the Coates' little terrace house in Victoria Road, Reading and among the items brought to Barnhill Road was a grandfather clock, once the property of my great-grandfather, Joseph Chapman, one time grocer in Wootton Bassett and latterly a clerk in the Huntley and Palmer biscuit factory in Reading. The clock was a brass-faced timepiece with the large initials 'T K' engraved among the figures and the works all assembled with tiny wedges or keys and a few rather crude screws. From the works were

161

suspended three wirelink chains where the ends of the wire in each link were merely butt-jointed so they could open up to drop one of the three heavy cast iron weights, each hung on a hook from a wooden pulley wheel in the bottom loop of each chain. Official inspection of the clock gave its age as 1680–1700 but the maker's initials 'T K' could not be traced and as the works were housed in a rather battered and obviously cheap case, it seemed likely that the original case had succumbed to the attentions of the insect world at some time in the life of the clock. When Barnhill Road was finally evacuated in 1960, disaster struck when the removal man put his arm round the clock case and lifted it bodily. The glass door over the face opened and the whole works, which were stood inside, fell out of the case on to the floor with unhappy results. The strike gong was cracked and of the eight chime gongs, five were shattered and will be irreplaceable as they were rough and rather irregular sand castings.

Diabetes had claimed a number of 'Nailers' over the years and in the 1950s Aunt Lil's condition deteriorated and she had one leg amputated. In 1958 she was admitted to the Royal Berks Hospital for the amputation of the second leg. I sat in the trike one Saturday morning outside No 78 when the telegram boy arrived and somehow I knew what it meant. It was from Ernie and it simply said 'Lilly died this morning'. I vowed to visit Ernie at Baughurst next day, but was thwarted by a petrol leak on the Morris 8.

Cyril Porter's disability and its associated problems got the better of him in 1961 and he died in Hammersmith Hospital and in January of that year we were summoned to North-wood to take sister-in-law Shirley up to Mount Vernon Hospital where Enid's brother was dying.

Brian was twenty five and swotting hard on accountancy, but nephritis overtook him and he succumbed a few days after his son's third birthday. They lived in an upstairs flat in Northwood Hills to which we took Shirley home after his demise. I climbed the stairs on my bottom and soon after that Shirley's mother arrived in some distress.

'Someone must stay with you,' she said and so it was that Enid volunteered us to spend a few nights at Northwood, Shirley eagerly accepted our offer to stay and the little boy looked a bit bewildered by it all, but seemed able to survive the message that his daddy would not be coming home again. The humping up and down stairs on my bottom was quite an effort and Enid and I would load into the A35 van early each morning, drive home to Charterhouse Avenue in Wembley, where I would transfer to the trike to set out for Victoria and Enid would walk to the station to take the train to Watford and Radiant House, a process to be reversed each evening. We kept this up for a whole week, whence Shirley seemed to be a little more settled, so we gave up this exhausting routine and returned home.

Immediate family seemed to be falling off fast and more was to come after our trip to Ireland in 1963.

We arrived home on Sunday evening and phoned my mother, to be told that my father was not at all well, so we tootled round to their bungalow in Kenton where it was obvious that my father had had a slight stroke. He took to his bed and a week later he was dead. After dealing with the immediate matters, I telephoned Baughurst to leave a message for Ernie, which brought a telegram to say he would be arriving at Paddington station on Saturday morning and indeed it was a great relief to see moral support right there in Kenton so soon after Dad's passing.

The rather stolid and staid presence of Ernie Evans was in itself a calming and reassuring factor and yet another example of the thought he always gave to other people's troubles and no more so than on the day of the funeral. The only other mourners would be my mother's two sisters and their husbands and they arrived a few minutes before the funeral left the house to head for Hoop Lane, Golders Green, where I chose for my father to be cremated. On return to Kenton, they had a quick cup of tea and decided they must depart despite the fact that I was looking to them for a little support for my mother at that particular moment. I was about to protest at their hurried departure, but Ernie restrained me and probably rightly so.

Enid's mother had already suffered a stroke but she struggled on over the years until our holiday in 1966, when we arrived in Abergele on the North Wales coast, there was a message to phone home. Enid's mother had died that day, so the following morning we packed up and returned home to deal with her father's problems and stayed the week to get him over the funeral. It was a great blow to Enid who was very close to her mother, but we returned to Abergele for the second week of our holiday.

The following year, when Ernie Evans was on one of his occasional visits to my mother in Kenton, he was overtaken by a stroke and admitted to Edgware General Hospital where, during his stay, I visited him each evening, an indication of the value of the trike as independent transport. When partially recovered he was mobile, but his speech was seriously affected when we took him back to Baughurst, where two of his sisters moved in to care for him. This arrangement lasted for a short time before he felt able to cope with his own needs and they returned to Reading.

I continued to take my mother and Enid to visit him at Stone Lodge for the joy of sitting in my chair in that peaceful garden and for the welcome he always managed to make clear to us, until 1968 when a message came from his sisters to say that Ernie had died in his bed at home. It was a sad moment for me and my memory went back over the past years of my life where Uncle Ernie had been a true friend in so many ways.

Cremation was at Henley, where they had spent their honeymoon in 1912 and my mother, Enid and I attended, but I have always regretted that I did not accept the invitation to return to his niece's home in Tilehurst after the funeral where so many of the folk I knew in those happy days at Broad Oak were gathered for a quiet cup of tea.

My mother continued to live alone in Kenton until the day near the end of 1972 when we were called to attend as she had fallen over in the street. The doctor came and persuaded her that she should come to stay at Charterhouse Avenue for a few days and then he told us privately that it was probably the end. We took her home but she became increasingly restive and the doctor had her admitted to Harefield Hospital from where the night sister rang up at 3 am one morning in December to say that my mother had died.

It was a great blow and I arranged the funeral at Hoop Lane Crematorium and had an entry made in the book of remembrance exactly as she had done for my father nine years before and each of those years on the anniversary of his death in July, we took my mother to the chapel to read again the entry that she had made, as it seemed to make her happy.

Our near relations were now very thin on the ground, leaving Enid's father as the last parent. He suffered advanced memory loss over the years and it was Enid's custom to phone him each lunchtime to check on his eating habits at midday, until the day that there was no reply. We headed for Bushey that afternoon and as we rounded the corner we observed that his curtains were drawn and the light was still on. Entering the bungalow we found him lying on the floor, having fallen from his chair the previous evening. The doctor pronounced him dead and the police were advised and proved most helpful with the arrangements from then on. After the funeral we sat back and looked around us – there were no near relations any more. Enid had a sister and a nephew, while I had two aunties and one cousin, brought about by a sequence of events.

Enid's nephew, Kevin, gained a stepfather when his mother, Shirley, married again and there were two children of that marriage, a son and a daughter, but when Kevin himself came to be married in 1984, I was prevented from attending by 'indisposition'.

That phenomenon of the age, the wedding video, had arrived by that time and prior to the ceremony, Shirley promised that I should see the video, but after the wedding, the months rolled by and no invitation came, until the evening I received a phone call when a faint croaky voice said, 'It's Shirley.'

The voice was unrecognisable and the story was sad, for she had been fighting off the advance of cancer since before the wedding. So next day we went to Northwood again to see a Shirley whom we could barely identify, following a course of chemotherapy, with customary results. It came as a great shock to me and my mind went back to the death of Brian all those years before.

In the midst of all this, one of my two remaining aunties was admitted to Westminster Hospital where regular visits began and the doctor duly informed me that she had a bladder growth. Her life became progressively more miserable as she returned home to her bungalow in Lancing, to be taken later into Southlands Hospital, where the end was obviously near. Twice the doctor had her shipped out to one of the myriad of nursing homes for the elderly that litter the south coast and twice it was an uncomfortable one night stay, as her condition was so poorly she could not be accommodated, other than in hospital. Such is the life of a lonely person – always the prey of the unscrupulous.

When it came to settling her affairs and disposing of the bungalow, my estranged auntie who had emigrated to the USA more than thirty years before, suddenly took an interest. A letter to the solicitor dealing with the deceased's affairs said, 'Don't sell the bungalow in the Fall, keep it till the Spring when the price will rise!' As the solicitor was not working for auntie on the thirty fourth floor of a skyscraper in New York, he dutifully ignored the letter and final settlement gave my cousin and myself one penny each more than auntie in America!

By Christmas 1986, Shirley was busy planning the wedding of her only daughter, Julie, the following July, but for Shirley it was not to be, for she died early in the New Year, to be buried with Brian in Northwood.

The wedding went ahead on 4 July, when Julie married her Prince Charming and it is to be hoped they will live happily ever after.

My father was an only child and so was I, while my mother was the eldest of five children, from whom there was but myself and one cousin. Of the Nailer side of the family with whom it was possible to keep in touch, there were no children. Ernie and Lily had no family and Violet, the only daughter of Uncle Alf, remained living in the Old Cottage in the Avenue at Bucklebury without ever marrying and of the other Nailers I have no trace, despite the thirteen children produced by my great grandfather, John Nailer.

In 1980, I had a strange telephone call from an Anthony John Nailer, living in Dorchester. It appeared that we were related just five generations back in the 1790s, where he was descended from one, Joseph Nailer, christened in 1768, while my own forebear was John, younger brother of Joseph, christened in 1772, at a time when parish records rated christening dates above birth dates. All were baptised in St Mary's Church at Bucklebury where the reverend gentleman must have been a very busy man in those days.

The family tree produced by Anthony John in 1986 from

very extensive research in many different record sources, took the line back to another John Nailer, born around 1700 and who married Hannah Ivey in Beenham in 1743.

The second of their three sons produced seven children within ten years, of whom the third son John had nine children, the eldest being William, christened in May 1799. William lies buried in Bucklebury churchyard under a cast iron headstone near the church door, but there is no sign of the resting place of his wife, Elizabeth Green, whom he married in 1823.

William's family of six children included one set of twins, but it was the eldest son, John, born in 1825, who married Mary Anne Wigmore on Christmas Eve 1856 and produced thirteen children, of whom my grandfather, Frederick, was the fifth. That leads on to the aforesaid tale in the text of which six of those thirteen children are mentioned, but the vine withers and from my end of the tree, that seems to be that!

EPILOGUE by his Wife

The wheel turns full circle

1989 had arrived – the year that the Middlesex group of the Disabled Drivers' Association celebrated forty years of active life in the community – a time for nostalgia, a time for celebration and a time for action!

Much thought and planning had gone into a more ambitious programme of group events than for many a long year, a programme in which Fred was prepared to participate to the full. January saw the circulation of a press release which he stage managed; February, a Sunday lunch for committee members and their spouses and a celebratory issue of the group's newsletter, *Mrs Frequently* with Fred as guest editor; March, a nostalgia evening when in addition to a display of photos and group memorabilia, he gave a much appreciated slide show of invalid vehicles of this century from his accumulated stock of transparencies. Having completed these duties in the early months, he was ready to enjoy the further events of the year to be organised by others.

April found him mildly distressed with a breathing problem, but a change of medication improved the situation and he was able to attend and enjoy the group's fortieth anniversary dinner at the Hilton National in Wembley at which we, as a couple, were presented by an anonymous well-wisher, with a pair of lead crystal tumblers engraved with the words 'Forty years DDA Service 1949/89.'

In May the breathing problems returned in greater intensity and juggling with the medication achieved no improvement, so that on 1 June he was admitted to the local hospital where little could be done and where he was incarcerated when the group held its fortieth anniversary birthday party. Later he transferred to the Phipps Unit in a South London hospital, a special unit dealing primarily with breathing and other problems of older polios, where it was recommended that he should spend his nights in a respirator or 'tank', the modern friendly name for what he could only still regard as a 'drinker' or an 'iron lung'.

The wheel had truly turned full circle after nearly fifty one years and it was to prove a traumatic experience for him, tempered only by the unbelievably wonderful constant care and prompt attention to every need by the nursing staff in this unit.

Great effort was made to introduce new medication that would suit both his breathing problem and his heart condition, but this did not meet with success and sadly he passed peacefully away on 12 July at the age of sixty two.

Despite his problems in those last six weeks, he was still ready and willing for his knowledge and experience to be used to benefit others. At the local hospital he spent an afternoon assisting with student doctors' tuition, at Phipps he advised another patient on mobility equipment and only the evening before his death, he was relating his medical history to a visiting foreign orthopaedic surgeon.

But as he said at the end of the last chapter 'from his end of the tree, that seems to be that!' His branch of the Nailer dynasty has ended, but surely with a modicum of satisfaction that his life has caused just a few ripples on the sea of disability.

Family tree of Frederick David Nailer
Compiled by Antony Nailer of Dorset
31 December 1986.

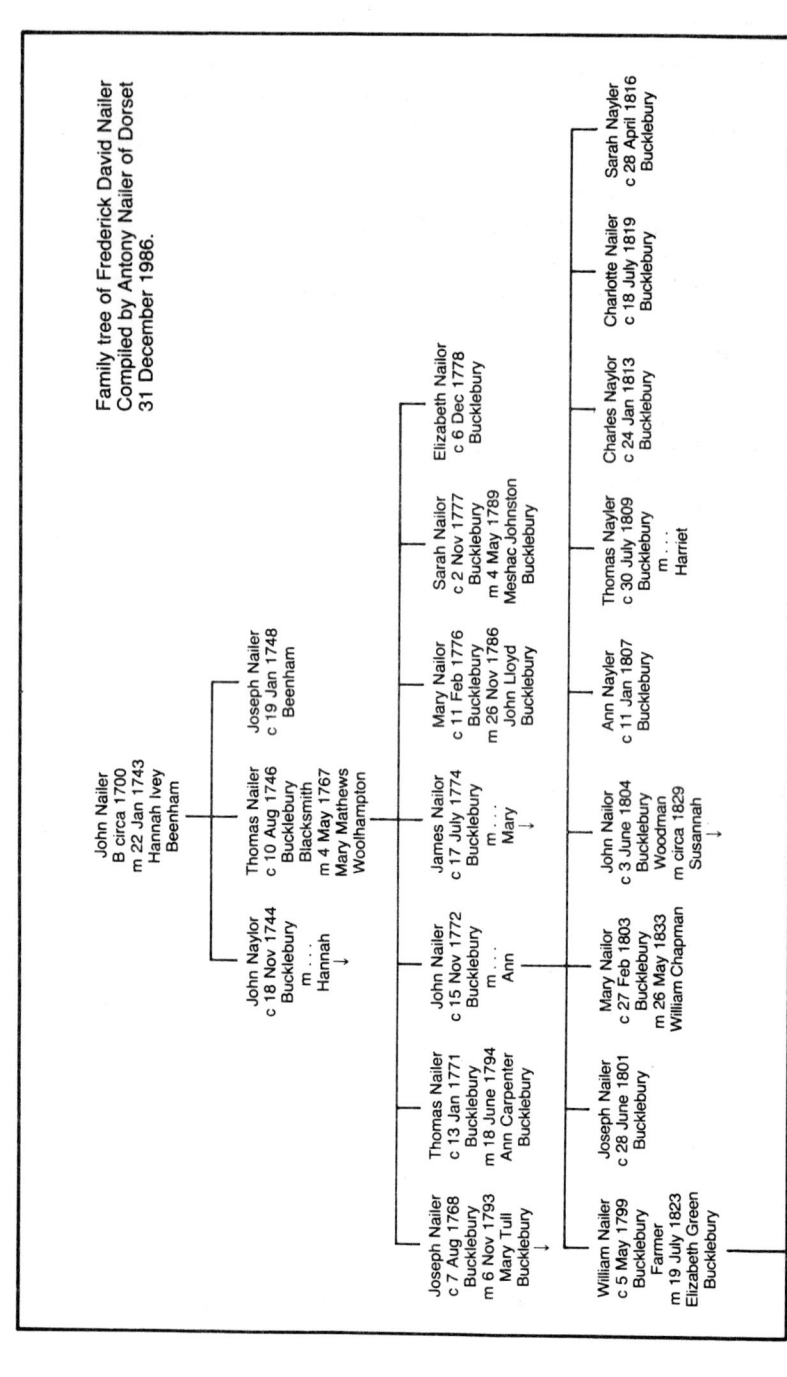

John Nailer
B circa 1700
m 22 Jan 1743
Hannah Ivey
Beenham

John Naylor
c 18 Nov 1744
Bucklebury
m . . . .
Hannah
→

Thomas Nailer
c 10 Aug 1746
Bucklebury
Blacksmith
m 4 May 1767
Mary Mathews
Woolhampton

Joseph Nailer
c 19 Jan 1748
Beenham

Joseph Nailer
c 7 Aug 1768
Bucklebury
m 6 Nov 1793
Mary Tull
Bucklebury
→

Thomas Nailer
c 13 Jan 1771
Bucklebury
m 18 June 1794
Ann Carpenter
Bucklebury

John Nailer
c 15 Nov 1772
Bucklebury
m . . . .
Ann

James Nailor
c 17 July 1774
Bucklebury
m . . . .
Mary
→

Mary Nailor
c 11 Feb 1776
Bucklebury
m 26 Nov 1786
John Lloyd
Bucklebury

Sarah Nailor
c 2 Nov 1777
Bucklebury
m 4 May 1789
Meshac Johnston
Bucklebury

Elizabeth Nailor
c 6 Dec 1778
Bucklebury

William Nailer
c 5 May 1799
Bucklebury
Farmer
m 19 July 1823
Elizabeth Green
Bucklebury

Joseph Nailer
c 28 June 1801
Bucklebury

Mary Nailor
c 27 Feb 1803
Bucklebury
m 26 May 1833
William Chapman

John Nailor
c 3 June 1804
Bucklebury
Woodman
m circa 1829
Susannah
→

Ann Nayler
c 11 Jan 1807
Bucklebury

Thomas Nayler
c 30 July 1809
Bucklebury
m . . . .
Harriet

Charles Naylor
c 24 Jan 1813
Bucklebury

Charlotte Nailer
c 18 July 1819
Bucklebury

Sarah Nayler
c 28 April 1816
Bucklebury

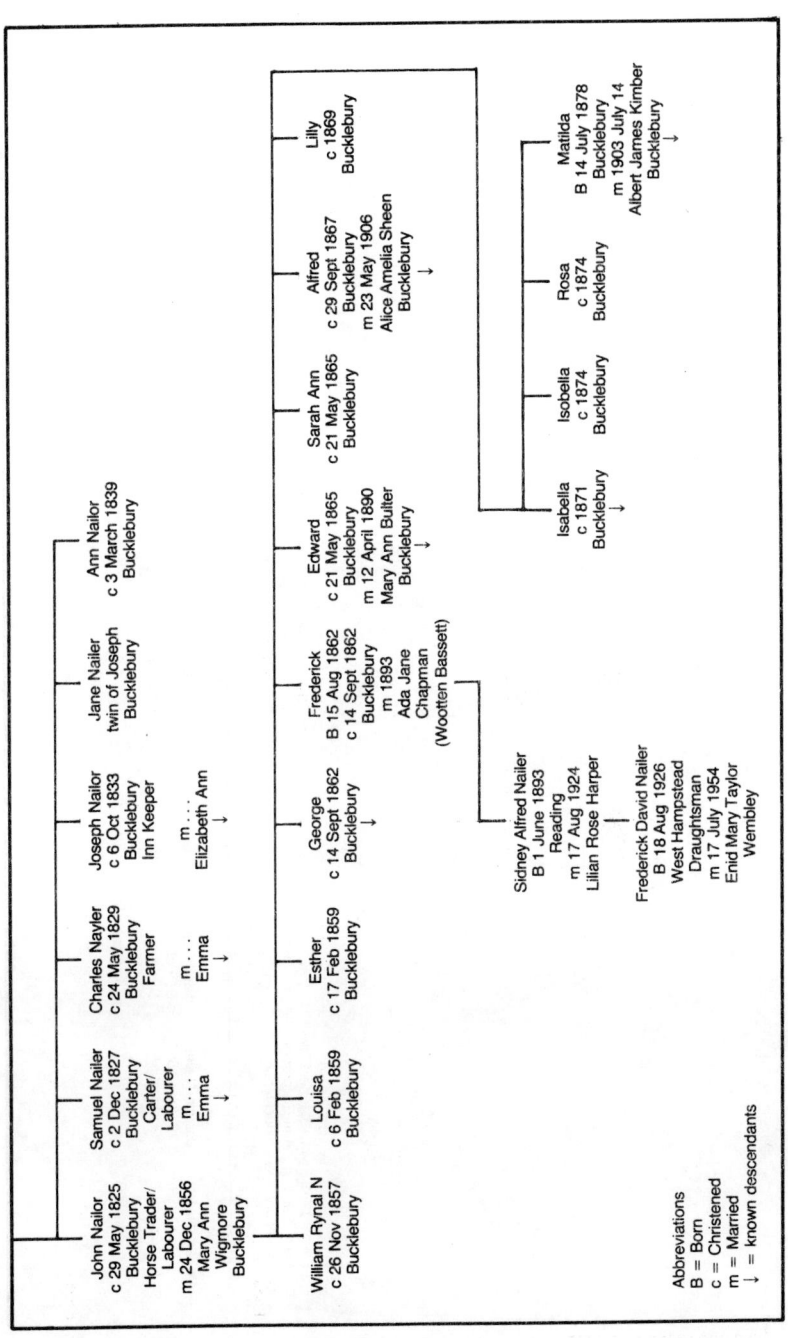

John Nailor
c 29 May 1825
Bucklebury
Horse Trader/
Labourer
m 24 Dec 1856
Mary Ann
Wigmore
Bucklebury

Samuel Nailer
c 2 Dec 1827
Bucklebury
Carter/
Labourer
m . . . .
Emma
→

Charles Nayler
c 24 May 1829
Bucklebury
Farmer
m . . . .
Emma
→

Joseph Nailor
c 6 Oct 1833
Bucklebury
Inn Keeper
m . . . .
Elizabeth Ann
→

Jane Nailer
twin of Joseph
Bucklebury

Ann Nailor
c 3 March 1839
Bucklebury

William Rynal N
c 26 Nov 1857
Bucklebury

Louisa
c 6 Feb 1859
Bucklebury

Esther
c 17 Feb 1859
Bucklebury

George
c 14 Sept 1862
Bucklebury
→

Frederick
B 15 Aug 1862
c 14 Sept 1862
Bucklebury
m 1893
Ada Jane
Chapman
(Wootten Bassett)

Edward
c 21 May 1865
Bucklebury
m 12 April 1890
Mary Ann Butler
Bucklebury
→

Sarah Ann
c 21 May 1865
Bucklebury

Alfred
c 29 Sept 1867
Bucklebury
m 23 May 1906
Alice Amelia Sheen
Bucklebury
→

Lilly
c 1869
Bucklebury

Isabella
c 1871
Bucklebury
→

Isobella
c 1874
Bucklebury

Rosa
c 1874
Bucklebury

Matilda
B 14 July 1878
Bucklebury
m 1903 July 14
Albert James Kimber
Bucklebury
→

Sidney Alfred Nailer
B 1 June 1893
Reading
m 17 Aug 1924
Lilian Rose Harper

Frederick David Nailer
B 18 Aug 1926
West Hampstead
Draughtsman
m 17 July 1954
Enid Mary Taylor
Wembley

Abbreviations
B = Born
c = Christened
m = Married
→ = known descendants